tremely interesting data and insights, and a useful understanding of the world of many teenagers in ten countries."

— From the Commentary by Harry C. Triandis, University of Illinois, Champaign, Illinois

Based on responses to a carefully translated, standardized self-image questionnaire, *The Teenage World* provides an opportunity to compare the self-images of large samples of adolescents in ten countries: Japan, Israel, Hungary, West Germany, Italy, Australia, Turkey, Bangladesh, Taiwan, and the United States. This is the first presentation of extensive data on cross-national differences in teenage self-image. The differences and similarities of self-image between older and younger teenagers, and between boys and girls are presented. Universal aspects of adolescent self-image are revealed as well as consistent cross-national gender differences and cross-national differences and demographic correlates of the adolescent experience.

Psychologists, psychiatrists, sociologists, social psychologists, and all professionals who encounter teenagers in their work will want to read *The Teenage World* to gain a better understanding of adolescent self-image throughout the world.

The Teenage World
Adolescents' Self-Image
in Ten Countries

The Teenage World
Adolescents' Self-Image in Ten Countries

Daniel Offer, M.D.
*Michael Reese Hospital and Medical Center
and Pritzker School of Medicine
University of Chicago
Chicago, Illinois*

Eric Ostrov, J.D., Ph.D.
*Michael Reese Hospital and Medical Center
Chicago, Illinois*

Kenneth I. Howard, Ph.D.
*Northwestern University and
Michael Reese Hospital and Medical Center
Chicago, Illinois*

and

Robert Atkinson, Ph.D.
*University of Southern Maine
Gorham, Maine*

With the collaboration of

Enrico de Vito, M.D. (Italy)
Muhammad Nazmul Haq (Bangladesh)
Banu İnanç, Ph.D. (Turkey)
Mária Kertész, M.D. (Hungary)
Shiroe Miura, M.D. (Japan)
Yukuhiko Miyoshi, P.S.W. (Japan)

Peter W. Musgrave, Ph.D. (Australia)
Sadao Ohshima, Ph.D. (Japan)
Amiram Raviv, Ph.D. (Israel)
Rachel Seginer, Ph.D. (Israel)
Hans-Christoph Steinhausen, M.D. (West Germany)
Sara Turner, M.A. (U.S.A.)

and with a commentary by
Harry C. Triandis, Ph.D.

Plenum Medical Book Company • New York and London

Library of Congress Cataloging in Publication Data

The Teenage world: adolescents' self-image in ten countries / Daniel Offer. . .
[et al.].
   p.   cm.
   Includes bibliographical references and index.
   ISBN 0-306-42747-8
   1. Self-perception in teenagers. I. Offer, Daniel.
BF724.3.S35T44 1988
155.5—dc19   88-4127
                                                  CIP

© 1988 Plenum Publishing Corporation
233 Spring Street, New York, N.Y. 10013

Plenum Medical Book Company is an imprint of Plenum Publishing Corporation

Printed in the United States of America

To Marjorie, Phyllis, and April
for the gift of love
 . . . Dan, Eric, and Ken

International Collaborators

Enrico de Vito, M.D.
Research Coordinator
Provincia di Milano
Centro di Psicologia Clinica
V. le Piceno, 60
Italy

Muhammad Nazmul Haq
Lecturer
Mymensing Teachers' Training
    College
Mymensing
Bangladesh

Banu İnanç, Ph.D.
Assistant Professor of Psychology
Çukurova University
Balcali-Adana
Turkey

Mária Kertész, M.D.
Specialist for Pediatrics and
    Adolescent Medicine
Orsó-utca 53
Budapest 1026
Hungary

Shiroe Miura, M.D.
Chairman, Department of
    Psychiatry
Tokyo Medical College
6-7-1 Nishishinjuko
Suginami-Ku
Tokyo
Japan

Yukuhiko Miyoshi, P.S.W.
Teacher of High School
Katoh-Gakuen High School
1979 Ohoka-Jiyugaoka
Numazu-city
Shizuoka Prefecture
Japan

Peter W. Musgrave, Ph.D.
Professor of Education
Monash University
Clayton, Victoria 3168
Australia

Sadao Ohshima, Ph.D.
Professor of Sociology and
    Psychology
University of Meiji-Gakuin
1-2-37 Shirogane-dai
Minato-ku
Tokyo
Japan

Amiram Raviv, Ph.D.
Professor of Psychology
Tel Aviv University
Ramat Aviv
Tel Aviv 69978
Israel

Rachel Seginer, Ph.D.
Assistant Professor of Education
University of Haifa
Mount Carmel
Haifa 31999
Israel

Hans-Christoph Steinhausen,
   M.D.
Acting Chairman, Department of
   Child Psychiatry
Freie Universität Berlin
Psychiatrische u. Neurologische
Klinik und Poliklinik
Platanenallee 23
D-1000 Berlin 19
West Germany

Sara Turner, M.A.
Professor of Sociology
Humboldt State University
Arcata, California 95521
(Taiwan research)

Acknowledgments

This study would not have been possible without the enthusiastic help of our collaborators, their students, and cooperating high schools. We thank them all, and hope that the results of our study will help us to better understand the citizens of tomorrow's world.

We are indebted to Ellen Mercer from the American Psychiatric Association, who helped us continuously and encouraged us during difficult days. Professor Marvin Zonis of the University of Chicago helped us in better understanding the vicissitudes of cross-cultural research. The following individuals helped us in back-translating the Offer Self-Image Questionnaire (OSIQ) to English: Dr. K. Lau, Dr. S. Contro, Dr. H. Kisisel, Dr. I. Kisisel, Ms. Pninah Zucker, Ms. Shiaomay Young, and Dr. M. Csikszentmihalyi.

The adolescent research fellows at Michael Reese Hospital have listened to results at different stages of the project and have given us excellent feedback and constructive criticism. We thank them all.

We also wish to thank the following individuals who read various chapters of the book and offered us most helpful comments: Ms. T. Offer, Mr. R. Offer, Dr. T. Brown, Dr. M. Sabshin, Dr. D. Hawkins, Dr. P. Barglow, Dr. M. Schaefer, and Dr. C. Strozier.

A number of individuals have been helpful in the analysis of the data: Ms. Sandra Wisniewski, Dr. Marc Zola, and Mr. Bruce Briscoe. Ms. Marie Allison helped with typing and organizing, and our research secretary, Ms. Merry Wilson, has been a tower of strength, patience, and understanding. We are indebted to all of them.

Mr. Irving B. Harris has been a most generous supporter of our project. He believed in us and through his financial help has made it possible for us to undertake this study. We are deeply grateful.

Daniel Offer
Eric Ostrov
Kenneth I. Howard
Robert Atkinson
Chicago, Illinois

Contents

Appendixes

CHAPTER 1

Introduction

A Cross-National Study of Adolescent Self-Image

Adolescence is not, as has been previously assumed, a developmental stage that was defined after the industrial revolution. There is substantial historical evidence to suggest that adolescence and youth, as a stage, was recognized by the ancient Romans, Greeks, and even Egyptians. The concept survived through the Dark Ages. In *Le Grand Propriétaire*, written in 1556, it is stated: "The third age, which is called adolescence, . . . ends in the twenty-first year . . . and it can go on till thirty or thirty-five. The age is called adolescence because the person is big enough to beget children. In this age the limbs are soft and able to grow and receive strength and vigor from natural heat" (Aries, 1962, p. 21).

The span of years devoted to adolescent development varies in different cultures and with different definitions. The term *adolescence* is no longer equivalent to *pubescence*. "Adolescence" is a psycho-social-biological stage of development that corresponds to changes in many areas which accompany the transition from childhood to adulthood.

The working definition of adolescence we use is the stage of life that starts with puberty and ends at the time when the person has attained a reasonable degree of independence from his parents. Once in high school or its equivalent, the vast majority of teenagers have already undergone the biological changes of puberty. At the end of high school, the process of separation from the family of origin continues, although this is obviously not an identical process in all countries.

Early adolescent studies characterized this developmental period

1

as one of *Sturm und Drang* (storm and stress). Clinical evidence suggested that idealism, altruism, rebellion against the established ways, and the expression of deep passions characterized the universal developmental psychology of adolescents. Hall (1904), whose influential work introduced this phrase, based his theories on his personal experiences and observations, and on his knowledge of the romantic 19th-century literature. He thought that it was typical for adolescents to oscillate between extremes of psychological functioning. Accordingly, the adolescent might feel happy and altruistic one day and depressed and egocentric the next. Hall later changed the German term *Sturm and Drang* to "adolescent turmoil."

Anna Freud (1958), from her extensive psychoanalytical experience with disturbed children and adolescents, expanded on this theme, emphasizing that the biological changes of adolescence are totally disruptive for the individual. Psychoanalytic theory concerning adolescent development still focuses on adolescent turmoil. Blos (1961) and, more recently, Rabichow and Sklansky (1980) characterized adolescence as consisting of impulsive behavior, mood swings, and introspection. Its hallmark, in short, is seen by these authors as a turmoil that abates only with the gradual strengthening of controlling, inhibiting, quieting, and evaluative principles, which takes place after adolescence. These theorists picture adolescents as attempting to function in the midst of an internal storm.

Adolescence has often been characterized as an in-between stage, when the boy is not quite a man and the girl is not quite a woman. It has been conceptualized as a unique transitional stage. Unless the personality undergoes major qualitative leaps in its organization, this view holds, maturation or adulthood cannot be achieved—stability or continuous, relatively uninterrupted growth is conceptualized as a failure to mature.

For over 20 years our research team has been investigating the psychology of normal adolescents. We have described how American middle-class teenagers cope with growing up: the kinds of psychological problems they have, how they deal with these problems, and how successful or unsuccessful they are in resolving their conflicts. We have described their psychological world, including their relationships with peers and family. A particular interest has been in discovering what kind of psychological conflicts are difficult for adolescents to resolve and how many adolescents have serious psychopathological problems (Offer, 1969; Offer and Offer, 1975; Offer, Ostrov, and Howard, 1981a; Offer, Ostrov, and Howard, 1984).

Our empirical studies of adolescents have not supported the "adolescent turmoil" views. In an effort to discover whether normal adolescents are severely stressed by emotional turmoil, we (Offer, 1969; Offer and Offer, 1975; Offer *et al.*, 1981a) have undertaken a number of studies of normal (i.e., school- or community-based) adolescent populations. These investigations were based on the premise that differences in theoretical formulations might be due primarily to differences in the populations being observed, since most of these formulations have been based on experiences with emotionally disturbed teenagers. We have found empirically that it is possible for many normal adolescents to integrate their new affective, cognitive, biological, and social experiences and still grow with relatively little disruption (Offer *et al.*, 1981a). It is clear that adolescence has unique features, as does every stage of life. Each stage in life brings new challenges and opportunities. But the changes each stage brings may be relatively easily incorporated into the basic personality structure.

We did find that a significant minority of the normative group studied (approximately 15%) describe themselves as depressed, anxious, emotionally empty, or confused. This figure is high and indicates that turmoil and maladaptation are a real part of many teenagers' lives. This subgroup of adolescents includes psychiatric patients, juvenile delinquents, those who deviate radically from their parents' social values, and possibly the specially gifted. Adolescents who experience turmoil most likely grew up in a confusing, emotionally empty, or hostile familial system. But these adolescents were far outnumbered by those who were relatively happy, coped well with their lives, and made a relatively smooth transition to adulthood.

The vast majority of adolescents report being relaxed under everyday circumstances. They believe they can control their day-to-day trials and tribulations without undue concern. Little evidence of mood swings, unpredictability of behavior, or deep-rooted cultural pessimism among these teenagers is found. The symptoms that were observed in these subjects were mild and situational in nature. When rebellious behavior was observed, it was relatively mild and it seemed most likely a function of achieving the initial step in the process of emancipation from the parents.

From these empirical studies, we concluded that adolescence does present the individual with a special burden, a challenge, and an opportunity. Adolescents have to individuate, establish self-confidence, make important decisions concerning the future, and free themselves from earlier attachments to parents. The majority of the teenagers in our studies coped with these tasks successfully. They lacked the turmoil of the disturbed adolescent precisely because their egos were strong enough to withhold the various pressures that they face in their lives. These subjects were not only well adjusted, they were in touch with their feelings and developed meaningful relationships with significant others, be they peers or parents.

The transition to adulthood is usually accomplished gradually and without undue upheaval. The findings of these empirical studies suggest emphatically that a state of turmoil need no longer be the password of adolescence. There are many current studies that report findings similar to our own: Block (1971), Douvan and Adelson (1966), Rutter, Graham, Chadwick, and Yule (1976), Vaillant (1977), Westley and Epstein (1969).

THE INTERNATIONAL STUDY

Our approach to studying adolescents cross-nationally is, in principle, the same as that used in our previous research; that is, it is necessary to evaluate adolescents' functioning in multiple areas, since an adolescent can master one aspect of his or her world while failing to adjust in another. In addition, we believe that the psychological sensitivity of the adolescent is sufficiently acute to enable us to obtain meaningful results by asking a teenager to respond directly to a set of standardized questions. For that reason, one of us (Offer) constructed the Offer Self-Image Questionnaire (OSIQ) 20 years ago. The experience that we have had with the OSIQ has convinced us that our approach to studying the psychology of adolescence with this test was warranted. The evidence indicates that the OSIQ is both reliable and valid. It has been utilized in hundreds of studies in the United States alone, and our data bank contains the results from over 30,000 adolescents.

In the early 1980s the OSIQ was translated into a number of different languages. It seemed to us that we had a unique opportunity to undertake a cross-national study that would help us discover what adolescents in different countries are feeling and thinking, how similar or different adolescents describe themselves in different countries, and what they have to tell us—adults—about their own psychological world.

In the spring of 1982 we wrote the following letter to investigators from 16 countries where we knew that translations of the OSIQ existed.

Dear Dr. _____:

We greatly appreciate the interest you have shown in the Offer Self-Image Questionnaire (OSIQ) and we would like to bring you up to date about our work with this instrument. We also invite you to participate in a new research project we are planning.

Our most recent OSIQ publication is a new manual (1981); we will mail this manual to you under separate cover in order to acquaint you with our new standard scoring and profile system. We are sending you several of our recent articles based on the OSIQ plus our book, *The Adolescent: A Psychological Self-Portrait* (Basic Books, 1981). The book is based on OSIQ results from thousands of adolescents from the USA.

The project we are inviting you to participate in is directed toward the assessment of the universality of the adolescent experience. We intend to collect samples of adolescents from many countries, using OSIQs translated into the language of each country.

For this project you could help us a great deal if you would provide us with completed OSIQs from a current representative sample of teenagers from your country. We would be glad to provide you with computer analyses, free of charge, of your data and to make these data available to you for your use and publication. We want to use your data for comparison with data from other countries. We would like a minimum of 100 subjects from each of the following four categories: younger (13- to 15-year-old) males, younger females, older (16- to 19-year-old) males, and older females.

Looking forward to working with you on this exciting project,

Sincerely yours,

Daniel Offer, M.D.
Eric Ostrov, J.D., Ph.D.
Kenneth I. Howard, Ph.D.

We were fortunate in obtaining the cooperation of investigators from nine countries: Australia, Bangladesh, Hungary, Israel, Italy, Japan, Taiwan, Turkey, and West Germany. With the addition of the United States, we had a sample of ten countries, which provide the data base for this book.

Investigators from seven other countries were unable to participate for a variety of reasons enumerated below:

USSR: The plans for the study, although agreed upon, were never consummated.

Holland and Ireland: The samples were too small to be included in the study.

France: The data arrived after our deadline passed.

Greece: It is our understanding that the study was completed, but we never received the data.

England and Switzerland: Although our colleagues wanted very much to participate, they were unable to get permission from the school systems in their communities.

This study is cross-national in design. Subjects in all the countries attended high school when they took the OSIQ. All belonged to the middle class. All were able to read and understand the various items in the OSIQ. Although the experience was more novel in Bangladesh than in the United States, the Bengali teenagers adapted well to the test-taking experience and said they enjoyed the experience.

The study was made possible, in large part, because communication of scientific results is increasingly international in scope. It is less and less true that studies are reported only in one language while investigators in other countries are unaware of the results. Consequently, the fact that our research was conducted in many languages is simply a sign of the times. Just as the industrial revolution forever changed the nature of the Western (and later non-Western) world, so the current communication revolution is changing the nature of the exchange of scientific information, making information instantly available all over the world. Satellites also have enabled people in different and geographically distant countries to experience similar events and to identify, at least in part, with similar universal phenomena affecting all people. An example is the near-universal witnessing of events such as space travel.

That revolution helped make our study possible. It is not only that our collaborators were able to select similar samples in the ten different countries, and that the data-collection phase took only 18 months; more dramatically, the psychological test that is the centerpiece of this study—which was written in English and standardized, validated, and shown to be reliable in the United States—was also shown to be a valid and reliable instrument in nine other countries (see Appendix 2). The vast majority of the teenagers found the psychological test meaningful and had no problems in responding appropriately.

Because of the ability to communicate so quickly anywhere in the world, the years since World War II have seen a continuous move toward decreasing cross-national differences or increasing universality of psychological experiences. We know, of course, that at the same time this movement toward universality has occurred, a cross-current of nationalism has arisen that stresses national differences. Both forces are hard at work. It is too early to decipher what shape society will have in the twenty-first century. Whether there will be a lessening or a strengthening of national differences we do not know. It seems to us, however, that as cross-national boundaries decrease, children and adolescents will know each other's world much better than ever before.

As we shall see in this book, adolescents growing up in very different countries are, on the whole, more similar to one another than they are different. No matter what the theoretical context in which they are embedded, these data present a unique international testimony—that of 5,938 adolescents, from ten diverse countries, letting us know what constitutes their psychological world.

Following this introduction, the book is divided into five chapters, dealing with theory, study method, results, discussion, and appendixes of the data. The *theory* chapter includes an extensive review of the literature on theories of the self in adolescence, cross-cultural studies of adolescents, and research issues in comparative studies. That on *method* describes our approach to data analysis and statistics, as well as a description of the ten countries where the study was undertaken. The *results* chapter contains our findings. We focus on the universal characteristics as well as on gender, age, and national differences. We also examine the prevalence rate of depression in the ten countries as well as the relationships of self-image patterns to economic and demographic factors. The *discussion* chapter integrates our findings with the current status of adolescent psychology, as well as raising a new agenda for the future. The *appendixes* contain the International OSIQ items (back-translated), their percent endorsements, and the alphas and means of the scales.

CHAPTER 2

Adolescents
Self and Culture

The Adolescent Self • *Toward Studying Adolescents across Cultures*

THE ADOLESCENT SELF

The term *self-image* implies an image of something. But an image of what? It is not easy to point to the self or specify exactly what the concept designates. Clearly, the self is a complex concept with multiple meanings. As one might expect, given this complexity, a review of the literature reveals a variety of views about the nature of the self. In this chapter, we shall elucidate the meaning of self from this variety of viewpoints, particularly as this concept applies to adolescents.

William James: The "I" and the "Me"

The *Oxford English Dictionary* (1933) defines self as "that which a person is really and intrinsically," having "successive and varying states of consciousness." This way of viewing the self recalls the original meaning of the Greek term *psyche*, connoting "animating force," "spirit," or "soul." Psyche literally referred to the essence of life. This standard definition of self and the original Greek term *psyche* both appear to point to what one is really seeking in self-knowledge: what it is that truly animates me; what it is that gives me my unique identity.

William James, who was perhaps the first self psychologist, pointed out that there are many selves. Particularly important is the growth and development of these selves throughout the adolescent years. These selves, optimally, eventually are integrated to form a total self from which a person draws a many-layered answer to the question Who am I? According to James (1890), each of the selves that constitutes the person has its own vulnerability, its own time of ascendancy, and its

9

own reason for being. The total self is a complex, fluctuating, expanding and contracting entity. In the widest sense of the term, one's self
includes all that can be called one's own. The self is one's body, psychological abilities, clothes, house, family, ancestors, and friends. It
also includes one's reputation, works, and emotions.

According to James, the self can be divided into three parts: (1) the
material self, (2) the social self, and (3) the spiritual self. The material
self consists of one's body, possessions, immediate family, and home.
The social self comprises the recognition one gets from others: one's
social identity, relations, roles, and reputation. James asserted that we
have an innate propensity to get noticed, and noticed favorably. "No
more fiendish punishment could be devised, were such a thing physically possible, than that one should be turned loose in society and
remain absolutely unnoticed by all the members thereof" (1890, p.
281). Within the spiritual self, James placed inner or subjective being,
as well as psychic faculties, dispositions, or states of consciousness.
These he saw as the most enduring and intimate part of the self.

With regard to the material self, during adolescence body image is
a critical concept. Bodily changes are rapid and symbolize the transition from childhood to adult status. Feelings about family are equally
important, coming in the context of the uniquely adolescent task of
forming a new relationship to parents and siblings while moving toward establishing one's own conjugal family.

James commented on a social-self phenomenon that may be very
prevalent among adolescents, when dealing with peers as well as other
groups in different situations. "It is his image in the eyes of his own
'self' which exalts or condemns him as he conforms or not to certain
requirements that may not be made of one in another walk of life"
(1890, p. 282).

The spiritual self is a vaguer concept. What is the spirit of adolescents? We have pointed out on other occasions that to many writers the
spirit of adolescents is one of turmoil and rebellion. Our view has been
very different (Offer, Ostrov, and Howard, 1981a). In this book we shall
attempt to assess that spirit as it is shown by teenagers in many countries throughout the world.

Sometimes, James noted, rivalry and conflict can exist among different selves. A teenager might say, "As teammates we play together to
win, but as students we compete for the best grades." We often have to
stand by one of our selves and relinquish the others. To be at once a
great athlete, excellent student, available and caring friend, creative
artist, proper son or daughter, and proper brother or sister is difficult, if
not next to impossible. If one were to try to achieve all these goals, a
number of different tensions would arise. James concluded, "The

seeker of his truest, strongest, deepest self must review the list carefully, and pick out the one on which to stake his salvation. All other selves thereupon become unreal, but the fortunes of this self are real" (1890, pp. 295–296).

The quest to develop harmony among selves is relevant to one of the central tasks of adolescence: identity formation (Erikson, 1950). The adolescent is more likely than the adult to have many selves competing for recognition and calling for potential integration. Adolescence is a time of trying out new roles, discarding or retaining old roles, and establishing a sense of coherence. A major goal of teenage development is to achieve a balanced, stable integration of selves that a teenager *cum* adult can own as "myself." Developing a balance and integration of selves is one of the hallmarks of the adolescent years. It is crucial, therefore, in examining adolescents' self-image, to take into account all aspects of the self.

James's conception of many selves also is pertinent because it is directly applicable to the structure of the questionnaire that was used in our study. That questionnaire measures the psychological self using impulse control, emotional tone, and body-image scales. It measures the social self—using social relationships, and vocational/educational goals scales—as well as the sexual self and the familial self. It measures the coping self using mastery of the external world, psychopathology, and superior adjustment scales. These five selves have counterparts in aspects of James's selves, particularly the material, social, and spiritual selves.

It should be pointed out that James's theory has important methodological implications for the study of the adolescent self. In a pioneering configuration, James divided the self into the "I" and the "me." The me is that aspect of the person that is known to or appreciated by the I. The I continually organizes and interprets experience. It is the me that is known to or appreciated by the person. Ordinarily, the acquisition of scientific knowledge consists of establishing replicable, consistent relationships between constellations of observations. Studying the self of another is inherently different from studying any other object or phenomenon because the self is a dual reality, both an I and a me. Most objects or phenomena consist of components that are observable and relatively invariant over time. In contrast, what one observes about another person is some combination of the I, the me, and the me presented by the I. An observer can never be sure which aspect of self is actually being observed. An inference about invariant characteristics of the I, the actor, may be a carefully inculcated persentation of the me. Or an observation of the me, the self-perception, could reflect a genuine attempt by the I to convey a perception of the self.

To gain scientific understanding of most phenomena, objective, systematic observations are usually enough. An alliance with the object of understanding is usually not needed. One does not have to elicit the active (intentional) cooperation of a thrown ball, for instance, to understand its trajectory. But often the best way to know another person is to ask that person about his or her self and to listen carefully to the answer. An alliance with the I of the other and empathic listening often will elicit more information relevant to knowing the other than any combination of unsolicited and unempathic observations of him. Only empathic listening in the context of another's willingness to reveal him- or herself will provide a key to the self of the other.

It is for this reason that in this book we understand the responses of our subjects as statements about themselves. We do so in contrast to viewing their statements as behaviors they emit in response to item stimuli. Our subjects' responses, we believe, are attempts to communicate about their selves, not just a set of behaviors to be catalogued. Our interpretations, therefore, will go to the issue of what these respondents meant to convey, and will not just represent a statistical compilation of them.

The Psychodynamic Adolescent Self

Adolescence, in a Freudian perspective, is a stage in a specific developmental process (S. Freud, 1949). To progress in a psychologically normal way, the young child must master sexual and aggressive drives in socially acceptable ways. The child must overcome competitive feelings toward the same-sex parent and sexual longing for the opposite-sex parent. Usually, young children accomplish these goals by identifying with the same-sex parent. They learn to satisfy yearning for admiration within the bounds of social acceptability. In the context of this line of development, adolescence represents a resurgence of sexual and aggressive drives. It also represents an awakening of conflictual feelings with respect to the parent of the same sex. There is an intensification of erotic feelings toward the parent of the opposite sex. Even if these longings and feelings were successfully mastered in childhood, the intensity of drives in adolescence tends to overwhelm old adjustments and create renewed turmoil in the teenage years (Blos, 1961). Adolescents, in this view, will almost always go through a protracted period of conflict and tumult. It could even be argued that an adolescent who did not go through conflict and tumult was not going through a needed transition and would fail to become a well-adjusted adult. Optimally, in the course of development the adolescent will learn to master drives and form a new, mature relationship with parents and other authority figures, paving the way toward successful adulthood.

Potential difficulties for adolescents include confusion and awkwardness about the body changes taking place in adolescence. Adolescents could be frightened or overwhelmed by their sexual feelings. They could fail to separate from parents or develop an extreme, rebellious attitude toward them. Some teenagers could try to master the tasks of adolescence through escape—for instance, through drug use or alcohol abuse. They could despair with respect to achieving adult goals and try to cope by withdrawal or even suicide.

Normal development would be indicated by a well-structured self-concept with stable, positive feelings about body, social relationships, and potential for accomplishment. Normal development includes age-appropriate sexual attitudes with non-conflict-ridden feelings and ways of behaving toward parents and peers of the opposite sex. From this point of view, in our terms, successful adolescence involves good adjustment in regard to body image, the sexual self, and the familial self.

One expression of a successful mastery of adolescent issues is the formation of a viable and coherent sense of personal identity (Erikson, 1950). Successful identity formation allows "the variety of changing self-images that have been experienced during childhood" (Erikson, 1982, p. 73) to be gradually brought into accord. Identity is the bridge between the individual and his society. A coherent and viable identity allows the individual to realize drives and longings in societally approved ways, while giving the individual a sense of meaningfulness and self-continuity. The danger for the adolescent is identity confusion, a failure to arrive at a consistent, coherent, and integrated identity. Identity confusion often is manifested as an inability to commit oneself, even in late adolescence, to an occupation or ideological position and to assume a recognizable station in life. While some identity confusion is considered to be "a normative and necessary experience," protracted confusion can lead to core disturbance and possible pathology (Erikson, 1982, p. 72). Another danger is a negative identity that involves "a debased self-image and social role" (Erikson, 1964, p. 97). Erikson has also discussed a less obvious problem, that of identity foreclosure or premature commitment to a social role.

A recent addition to the psychodynamic approach is that of Kohut (1985). This approach sees the self as the center of initiative, characterized by assertiveness and the power to form goals. The link to psychodynamic formations is that the self is shaped at its core by childhood influences that largely remain unconscious. As with James, Kohut's system includes many selves. Although there are conscious as well as unconscious selves, the one experienced by the individual as the most basic is the nuclear self. This is the self that controls not only the individual's most enduring values and ideals but also his or her most deeply anchored goals, purposes, and ambitions. The nuclear self has the capacity for introspection and empathy. The adolescent will approach life with a basic program, a plan for the future, and an anticipation of particular fulfillments. This basic program is largely a function of the nuclear self. Success for the adolescent will encompass developing a nuclear self that has reasonable narcissism, that is, self-valuing that is neither too demeaning nor unrealistically grandiose. With moderate narcissism, the self will be able to strive in a realistic way without falling prey to the twin dangers of trying to accomplish too much and thereby accomplishing nothing, or failing to strive at all in order to preserve a fragile self-appreciation.

Adolescence from a psychodynamic view, in short, begins with childhood (or even infantile) issues. Its focus is upon struggles with a resurgence of sexuality and aggression on the one hand, and longings and competitive feelings toward parents on the other. Adolescence ends with a focus upon more mature issues, such as trying to find an acceptable role in society, which involve reasonable ways of feeling good about oneself and trying to make self-fulfilling, realistic choices with respect to a spouse and the possibility of procreation.

The Adolescent as Authentic Self

The cognitive changes undergone by the teenager, along with the earlier physiological changes of puberty, constitute what Jung referred to as a "psychic revolution." The adolescent is beginning to open up not only to the personal self but to a collective realm as well.

For Jung (1959), the self includes an unconscious as well as a conscious component. Since the self is also the central archetype of the collective unconscious, it acquires certain universal characteristics. Jung (1961) actually viewed the self as the goal of psychic development. It is the principle archetype of orientation and meaning, of unity and totality, of order and organization; it is the essence of psychic wholeness, which unites the personality.

As Jung explained, there is "the premonition of a centre of personality, a kind of central point within the psyche, to which everything is related, by which everything is arranged, and which is itself a source of energy. The energy of the central point is manifested in the almost irresistible compulsion and urge to become what one is, just as every organism is driven to assume the form that is characteristic of its nature, no matter what the circumstances. This centre is . . . thought of . . . as the self. Although the centre is represented by an innermost point, it is surrounded by a periphery containing everything that belongs to the self—the paired opposites that make up the total personality. This totality comprises consciousness first of all, then the personal unconscious, and finally an indefinitely large segment of the collective unconscious whose archetypes are common to all mankind" (1959, p. 357).

For Jung (1933), this lengthy process of development toward the self begins sometime after puberty but, as our life's goal, is usually not fully effected until well into maturity. What was important for Jung is that the more one knows oneself, the more one will know of the world. The more the self is able to enter into the realm of the collective unconscious, the more the self becomes open to all the world. This new openness comes at the same time as the adolescent's interest in the social realm emerges.

The Adolescent as Social Learner

Social-learning theorists (e.g., Bandura, 1977) describe adolescent development as a product of social influences. Adolescents learn in an instrumental way—that is, their behavior is shaped by rewards and punishments resulting from specific behaviors experienced in conjunction with specific social milieus. Adolescents also learn from imitating others who serve as models for them. As time passes, adolescents achieve a view of self that incorporates the rewards, punishments, and modeled behaviors they have learned. Ideally, the view of self that teenagers have is consistent and adaptive. Having a consistent and adaptive self-image allows adolescents to achieve substantial self-control since, when confronted with a problem, they can see themselves as participants and effectively consider ways to cope with the problem rather than merely be reactive to it.

Bandura's theory lends itself particularly well to understanding the critical role of peers in adolescent development. In our terms, Bandura's theory is most pertinent to the social self. One of the most important tasks of adolescence is gaining psychological distance from one's family of origin and forming interpersonal bonds with peers. Teenagers reach out to and are heavily focused upon others in their age group. As a result, much of their self-formation occurs in the context of relationships with other teenagers. They imitate and learn from one another. Imitation, at the same time, does not preclude the development of unique individual standards and views. The influence of peers will be received in the context of unique values a teenager has acquired from, and the powerful ongoing influence of, his or her family of origin.

Evidence shows (Offer, 1969) that despite strong peer influence, the normative adolescent has not forgotten what was learned in the context of the family. Eventually, normal adolescents achieve a balance between the values and attitudes of friends and family. They attain a self that can be recognized as their own, one with which there is a sense of comfort.

Mischel's theory (1977), however, cautions us not to reify the self that is observed in any one context. That self represents an accretion of learning in specific social contexts. Consequently, the self is as much a product of the situation one finds oneself in as a product of disposition and tendencies that are present across situations. An adolescent's self will be coherent and persistent insofar as having a self with those qualities is rewarding to or viable for that adolescent. When, in a certain situation or context, these qualities cease to be rewarding or viable, a very different self might be observed. In our terms, we should remember that our questionnaire taps a multidimensioned reflective self that captures the usual experience of the teenager. In a radically different specific context, a different self might be observed, and we simply have to concede that our study does not encompass these other potential selves.

The Adolescent as Philosopher: Stages and Cross-Cultural Perspectives

Reflection upon one's self is implied in Plato's admonition "Know thyself." After the enlightenment, the Descartes dictum "I think, therefore I am" reflected an emphasis on consciousness. Today we are in the midst of a cognitive revolution wherein the self is viewed in part as an information-processing system. Reflecting the age of the computer, one view of the self is that it is made up of memories, processors, switches, and controls performing operations to compute new representations and thereby to manage its affairs in the world (Newell, 1985).

All cognitivists recognize that adolescents acquire greater reasoning and problem-solving capacity than they had as children. Turnbull (1983), an anthropologist drawing upon research spanning four continents, averred that youth is a time given to developing the art of reason, or the art of correct application of knowledge. It is through experiencing life fully, and joining this to the wholeness of knowing, he stated, that youth is able to find wisdom. Thus, the maturing teenager becomes a philosopher of sorts, turning bits and pieces of acquired knowledge into wisdom.

While it seems almost self-evident that wisdom increases during adolescence, a less obviously correct assertion is that cognitive abilities undergo a qualitative and irreversible shift during these years. A qualitative shift in cognitive abilities would involve adolescents' not only knowing more or thinking faster than children, but knowing and thinking in qualitatively different ways than children do. An irreversible shift would mean that once adolescents achieve this putative qualitatively higher form of cognizing, they cannot slip back into the lower, more childlike, form again.

Stage Theorists

Perhaps the most influential cognitive theorist is Piaget (1970). Piaget's work is structurally oriented. For Piaget, structures are whole systems that are subject to transformations and capable of self-regulation. The elements of such systems are subordinated to laws, and therefore self-maintaining in that the transformations inherent in a structure always tend to preserve the essential system. Piaget's structuralism differentiated between the individual subject, who is not of concern, and the epistemic subject—that cognitive nucleus which is common to all subjects at the same level.

Piaget's approach has been to understand the nature of knowledge and the structures and processes by which it is acquired. Piaget's studies (1967) indicated that mental development begins with no definite differentiation between the self and the external world. The self at this stage is the center of reality since it is not aware of itself. From ages 2 to 7, the child, through language, can reconstitute past actions, anticipate future actions, and represent itself intuitively. Ages 7 to 12 mark the period when the child is liberated from intellectual egocentricity. The child becomes capable of new coordinations, new moral feelings, and an organization of will that culminates in a better integration of the self. The older child is capable of more effective regulation of affective life.

By adolescence, Piaget says, egocentricity is present but occurs in the context of self-reflection. The Piagetian self, therefore, experiences three important decentralizations: sensorimotor, concrete, and formal. The third of these, completed in adolescence, enables one to reason about the world and the self using a formal operational thought process by which implications can logically be drawn from many related propositions.

To Piaget, adolescents are capable of combining thought processes into self-reflection about vocational goals, personal satisfaction, and social responsibility. Having reached the level of formal operations, teenagers can begin to philosophize. Maturing adolescents can utilize whatever innate or acquired knowledge they have, as well as newly developed capacities for logic, orderly analysis, and reflection. They thereby give greater cohesiveness and meaning to experience. For Piaget, mental life evolves toward a final form of equilibrium. The self becomes a true personality as self-reflective thoughts and feelings are integrated into a total life perspective.

Recent cognitive work relevant to adolescents has been carried out by Kohlberg and Gilligan (1971). These authors have described the relationship between cognitive and moral development in adolescence. To Kohlberg and Gilligan, cognition and moral reasoning involve schemata, or structural characteristics, which represent successive forms of psychological equilibrium. Justice, the equilibrium of affective and interpersonal schemata, has many of the same basic structural features as logic, the equilibrium of cognitive schemata. Moral judgments, and their development through stages, are an interdependent component of cognitive developmental stages. Formal operational thought, or cognitive maturity, is a necessary but not a sufficient condition for principled morality.

In Kohlberg's (1981) theory, there are three qualitatively separate levels of moral understanding, levels he called preconventional, conventional, and postconventional. These levels are irreversible in the sense that once one has achieved a higher level of understanding it is virtually impossible (except in extreme circumstances) to function at a lower level. The postconventional level is first evident in adolescence. This level is characterized by an autonomous, reflective perspective on societal values and the construction of moral principles that are universal in application. Gilligan (1982) noted that the factors shaping women's moral judgment, as well as their definition of the moral domain, differ from those of men. For women, the moral problem is seen as one of care and responsibility in relationships rather than as one of rights and rules. Thus, there is a logic of relationships operating among women, while a formal logic of fairness seems to inform the male approach to justice. This distinction between two modes of reasoning may contribute to the gender differences that are found among teenagers.

The adolescent as philosopher underlines the fact that adolescence is a time of growing cognitive ability and awareness. Those preteens who are by and large reactive to the world around them become self-reflective, often self-conscious teenagers. The consciousness of the teenager includes more clearly and coherently than ever an emotionally salient entity, namely, his or her own self. Adolescents develop the capacity not merely to memorize or recite ideas but to think about them. One idea they can think about is their own self.

In this book, the adolescent as philosopher is studied by asking about various moral values. The developmental approach of Piaget, Kohlberg, and Gilligan emphasizes the importance of distinguishing between younger and older adolescents, a distinction that is underlined throughout this book. It is during the later teen years, for instance, that one's capacity for an expanded world view most strongly comes into play. Gilligan's work makes clear the critical importance of gender to any psychological study. For this reason, in this book gender differences in self are a particular focus of interest.

One implication of Piaget for this work is that adolescents are particularly suitable as subjects for a study of the self. Adolescents are able to think about themselves and are motivated to do so. They can and want to introspect about themselves along many dimensions. Asking adolescents about themselves is an age-appropriate and particularly rewarding endeavor.

The Many and the One: Individual and Culture

Berger and Luckmann (1966), Goffman (1959), and Kelly (1955) represent the social-constructionist approach to the self. Personal constructs, social reality, and self-presentations are to a large degree shaped by our culture and, more specifically, our interactions with others. From this view, a heightened level of social interchange, in a particular cultural matrix, determines how adolescents view themselves. Anticipating one's social future, assuming new social roles, and becoming part of the dominant culture are all factors in adolescent self-image.

Kelly (1955) postulated that a person's thought processes seek to predict events in the real world. The self is therefore fundamentally oriented toward the future, tending to anticipate events by construing or interpreting one's role in the world. Like persons at any stage of development, adolescents look at themselves as an object to enhance the predictability of the world. What is usually anticipated is the reactions of others to one's self in a variety of contexts. Kelly's theory builds bridges to theories of culture. Because personal constructions of events differ, people differ. To the degree that two people employ a similar construction of experience, their psychological processes resemble each other. Since people belonging to the same cultural group tend to construe their experience in similar ways, culture has its influence in making constructs more similar among than between groups of people. From this perspective, the self of the adolescent can be seen as a function of both individual differences and cultural commonalities. Central questions for adolescents are: How am I different from others in my cultural group? How am I the same as others in my group? How do and will others react to me? How will I react to them in various circumstances? What do these reactions mean regarding who I am? The answers, provided by peers, culture, and unique individual experiences, will in large measure constitute the adolescent's self.

Another social-constructionist perspective is offered by Berger and Luckmann (1966). These authors saw the formation of the self as occurring through the interrelationship of organismic development and the socialization process. Both self and others are performers of objective, recurrent, and known actions. The socialization of the self includes assuming roles and internalizing independent phenomena that are found in one's world. One's self-image is determined by reactions to the social actions one is engaged in.

Adolescents, Berger and Luckmann teach us, cannot be understood apart from their social role and the social groups they interact with. Whom these adolescents perceive themselves to be will to a degree be a function of the groups they participate in. Group members' responses will change how they view themselves; those responses will lead to a qualitative change in who they are. It is not just that teenagers' behavior changes depending upon whom they are with. Who they are fundamentally and qualitatively will change as a function of what others perceive them to be and who, as a result, they perceive themselves to be.

Another approach to the adolescent in a cultural context is Goffman's (1959). Goffman emphasizes the concept of self-presentation. In his view, the self is an actor in a drama, with the individual as playwright and the persons with whom he or she is interacting as audience. The "performed self" attempts to present an image of itself that it would like others to hold. The crucial concern is whether the self-image that is presented will be credited or discredited by others. One role of culture is to teach what is and what is not generative of positive regard.

Goffman's work emphasizes the importance of image-making in the self put forward by an adolescent. Adolescents, Goffman implies, present both to themselves and to others. The adolescent self an outside observer sees is a complex product of an attempt by the adolescents to shape a self that is acceptable both to themselves and to others, as well as an attempt to accurately share their own "me." What they present is influenced by culture in three ways: culture affects what they are, it affects what they perceive themselves to be, and it affects how they portray themselves.

While the self is an evolving, changing, even elusive entity, its study in adolescence is enhanced by adolescents' attaining sufficient reflective awareness to arrive at a cohesive sense of self. Cultures differ. But all enhance the individual's ability to view personal feelings and experiences within the context of its interpretive schemes and symbols (Gardner, 1985). Through a combination of one's own intellectual competences, and through the interpretive schemes furnished by one's culture, it is possible to put forth a description of oneself that fairly well summarizes one's existence. With empathy and awareness of cultural differences, our premise is that an adolescent's self can be appreciated, even across the gulf of wide cultural differences.

Cross-Cultural Approaches

From a linguistic approach, Chomsky (1957, 1980) saw the self as based upon a preprogrammed knowledge of the underlying rules of structural principles common to all languages. This parallels the sociobiological view that social behaviors are genetically preprogrammed in the human species. Chomsky therefore hypothesized the existence of certain universals in the developmental process of learning a language. Children have an innate knowledge of these linguistic universals, and that enables them to learn in a standard sequence a complexity of tasks leading eventually to an infinite number of possible sentences.

There are substantive universals (based on descriptive groups) and formal universals (based on generative rules) in language as well as universal constraints that restrict the range of possible rules. According to Chomsky (1975), these universal constraints actually facilitate the learning process. He asserted that the surface structure (the phonetic sounds) varies, while the deep structure (the logical syntax) of all languages is similar.

This view raises some very interesting questions regarding the self. Can we make such a leap concerning the acquisition of self-knowledge, as Chomsky has with language acquisition? Can we say that an innate knowledge of social universals is a part of each person's birthright, that there are deep as well as surface universals regarding the self, and that there are universal constraints that restrict the range of one's social responses?

Chomsky's view provides clues regarding the study of the adolescent self across cultures. If there is a deep structure to the self of all persons, then a person from any one culture should be able to generate a frame of reference for understanding the self of persons in other cultures. In large measure, this book is premised on this implication from Chomsky. We have taken a structure—psychological self, social self, familial self, sexual self, coping self—and used it to assess the selves of adolescents in various countries throughout the world. The success or failure of such an endeavor can be seen as a test of this implication from Chomsky.

A theorist who is pertinent in this regard is Levi-Strauss (1966). Levi-Strauss was concerned, from the perspective of an anthropologist, with social structures and the manner in which they are learned by members of society. Focusing on conceptualizations of the structure of one's world, he argued that there is no fundamental difference between the traditional mind and the modern mind. Both use the same operations, both are capable of an advanced type of logic, but each applies them to different situations. Thus, he attempted to unify the mental structures of primitive and civilized peoples.

The Levi-Strauss program, by focusing on the mind, was designed to bring out the nature of a human psychology as well as social and cultural organization. This perspective has particular relevance for our study, not only for its inherent notion of intrahuman commonalities, or universals, but also because it implies that an instrument such as the OSIQ, designed originally for use by teenagers in a specific culture, could also be used by teenagers from very different cultures.

Summary of the Adolescent Self

What we recognize as the focus in almost all the literature just reviewed is that which animates the self. It appears that contemporary self theorists, though they might not admit it, are still looking at the self as psyche or soul. They are still concerned with what guides and inspires, directs and motivates the self. There may be no way to avoid this. The guided, inspired, directed, and motivated reflective is what teenagers from all over the world might have in common.

Chomsky and Levi-Strauss, though they start from different premises and are concerned with different intellectual problems, are the most notable proponents of the psychic-unity thesis in our time (Spiro, 1984). Jung, too, would have to be put in this camp. We are aware that juxtaposing the universalist and relativist viewpoints presents inherent problems. However, it is not always necessary to hold exclusively to one or to the other. Our view is that it is more realistic to acknowledge that there are some things you cannot understand about others, some things that are fundamentally different (relativism), while there are some things persons from all cultures can understand, that represent similarities among all peoples (universalism). The task is to know when it makes sense to emphasize the likenesses or the differences.

As socializers, adolescents are most concerned with social relationships, particularly in establishing friendships and developing a capacity for empathy with others. As cognizers, they struggle to understand the world in rational, coherent ways. In our terms, adolescents develop a self-concept and, in particular, a social self. In developing new feelings about parents and siblings, they shape a familial self. Their quest for new understanding affects their coping self. These selves evolve in the context of what actually is a lifelong quest, shaping and finding an answer to the question Who am I? It is in these areas that we posit universal themes and the bases for a common understanding.

As we identify the commonly held beliefs and values of our global sample, we begin to see the ways in which teenagers around the world think, feel, and behave similarly, leading us to posit aspects of a universal self-image. We see the process of becoming an adult as universal, as one that enables the world's teenagers to hold similar thoughts, values, and goals as they gradually arrive at a mature self-image, made up of similar and commonly experienced components. At the same time, qualitative differences will exist on such bases as gender, age, nationality, and culture. It is the quest to provide an empirical basis for these speculative commonalities and differences to which this book is devoted.

TOWARD STUDYING ADOLESCENTS ACROSS CULTURES

How is it possible to demonstrate "universals" or differences among adolescents from different countries and cultures? The history of cross-cultural comparative research is replete with examples of biased reports and methodological conundrums. Early studies, most notably the accounts of explorers and missionaries, carried a biased perspective that assumed cognitive differences, specifically the mental inferiority of "primitive" peoples. Some early anthropologists, particularly Boas, rejected such explanations of cultural differences, but the field still struggles today to overcome a bias based on the idea of higher and lower levels of culture. The purpose of this chapter is to provide a background for a comparative—in the ideal, unbiased—approach to psychology. This background will enable us to evaluate the extent to which adolescents from different countries can be validly compared to one another.

In our study we attempted to avoid some pitfalls by using subjects who came from similar social class backgrounds. Meaningful intergroup differences still could emerge on the basis of such factors as (1) culture and its impact on views and interpretations of social and physical phenomena, and (2) economic and demographic variables such as gross national product and population density. Because we looked only at countries with a viable middle class, the study of societies unaffected by modern technology is not an issue for us. All our subjects were literate and came from countries engaged in cultural and economic transactions with technologically developed nations. Our urban, middle-class subjects are likely to have been exposed to the

cultures and products of other nations. By using relatively sophisticated subjects who could cooperate with a research study such as this
one, we maximized comparability. In so doing, we took the position
that investigators from any culture can understand teenagers from other
cultures using standard instruments, given relatively minimal amount
of shared knowledge and understanding. The following survey of methodological issues explains the premises upon which this position rests.

Definitions

The self is a key construct of psychology; culture is a key construct
of anthropology. Ever since the two disciplines discovered each other,
debate over joint terminology, definitions, and scope has ensued.
Culture, like the self, is a term with many definitions, each corresponding to one aspect of what is a multifaceted concept. On the one hand,
culture is seen as a process (the passing on of what has been learned
before to succeeding generations) that involves concrete artifacts and
specific technological knowledge. On the other hand, culture can be
viewed as primarily involving shared meaning and symbol systems
(D'Andrade, 1984). A parallel distinction has been made between physical culture, such as material objects, and subjective culture, such as
people's attitudes, values, and beliefs (Triandis, 1972). It was Geertz
(1973) who perhaps most clearly brought all of these elements together
in one definition. He stated that culture denotes a system of inherited
conceptions expressed in symbolic forms and transmitted through a
pattern of meanings by which people communicate, perpetuate, and
develop their knowledge about and attitudes toward life.

What is called "cross-cultural" (Berry, 1980) in the social sciences
is referred to as comparative in other disciplines. The comparative
method is the core of the scientific method; without comparison, differences and similarities, covariation and cause cannot be observed or
inferred. When psychology uses cross-cultural methodology, it ideally
involves "the collective efforts of researchers who work among people
who speak various languages, live in societies ranging from technologically unsophisticated to highly complex and industrialized, and
who live under different forms of political organization" (Triandis and
Brislin, 1984, p. 1006).

"Cross-cultural" appears to describe our study quite well, since we
studied adolescents' psychological functioning in different countries.
In many circles, however, the term cross-cultural connotes work done
in "unsophisticated" or traditional societies. This is just the implication we want to avoid, since our subjects all come from industrialized,

urban settings. To make our position as clear as possible, it should be kept in mind that we use the terms *culture, nation,* and *society* interchangeably to describe the nature of our study.

A major premise of this book is that urban teenagers throughout the world are able to draw upon inner resources to reflect upon their self-image and experience. When teenagers reflect on statements such as "A job well done gives me pleasure," "I like to help a friend whenever I can," or "My parents are ashamed of me," it can be assumed that they draw upon knowledge they share with others within their particular meaning system. They also draw upon their individual attitudes toward life. Our premise is that these questions also tap a universal experience, that the answers can be viewed from a common reference point. We presume a Bengali teenager can assess her willingness to help a friend just as a Turkish youth can, that a Hungarian teenager can attest to or deny taking pleasure in work, using a subjective reference point comprehensible to an American teenager. In a sense, the data presented in this book constitute the evidence for this position. Our primary findings involve commonalities among adolescents from many different nations. As we hope to show, dimensions of selfhood devised to allow American teenagers to describe themselves were meaningful to teenagers in countries scattered around the globe.

Cross-Cultural Methodology

Any major contribution to the field of comparative psychology must take into account the variability of culture across human populations. It also must take into account the variety of human behavior found within a specific culture. Comparative studies have covered a wide range of topics and concepts central to psychology. Those studies generate two primary concerns.

First, cross-cultural psychology has no accepted guided theory (Triandis, 1980).Part of the reason for this, according to Lambert (1980), is that there are two equally viable and opposing theories: One emphasizes the "psychic unity of mankind," while the other reflects an extreme relativism in which few similarities in psychic functioning are expected. Second, cross-cultural research involves many methodological approaches (Brislin, 1983); cross-national studies are carried out by investigators of various disciplinary backgrounds, making it a field with no common core training.

These concerns can be addressed through considering the goals of cross-cultural or multinational research. These goals center around expanding the range of variability in human behavior studied by psychology, detecting uniformities and consistencies in structure and function across mankind, and checking the generality of existing psychological theory and laws (Berry, 1980).

Comparative Studies versus Cultural Relativism

A beginning point for discussion is Triandis's (1980) view that establishing cultural differences is extremely difficult. The strategy he advised was to give top priority to the establishment of the generalizability of psychological laws. It is essential to begin by establishing frameworks of similarity within which differences can be interpreted. The key methodological guidelines for the future call for researchers to provide integrative positions that focus upon the universal and involve psychologists from a wide variety of cultures in order to move more effectively toward psychological generalizations (Lambert, 1980).

Brislin (1983) made the point that optimally more collaborative efforts, in which data are gathered in many countries and shared among a number of collaborators, are needed. He felt it important to obtain input from members of different cultures concerning the concepts to be investigated and the methods to be used, as well as their reactions to a study's findings as soon as those findings are made. A study performed using this methodology could contribute greatly to cross-national psychological research. It was with these points in mind that we designed and analyzed our study.

Benefits of Comparative Studies

Comparative analysis, which allows general (or universal) statements about relationships among variables to be asserted, has the following advantages:

Theory Expansion

Theories usually stem from a limited set of observations tested only in the country of origin. Piaget's theory of cognitive development is an example. He began by making theoretical assertions based on his observations of Swiss children. He identified a four-stage process by which intellectual development occurs through childhood and into early adolescence. But his limited sample raised the fundamental question of the invariance of this process across cultures. Piaget (1973, p. 300) acknowledged that a solution to this problem "requires extensive cross-cultural studies." Only when a hypothesis is tested in various parts of the world—among people of various ethnic and social backgrounds—can that hypothesis be tested in its fullest sense. Only then has it met the rigorous test of comparative analysis (Triandis and Brislin, 1984).

Increased Range of Variables

Cross-cultural research is often used to obtain a wider range of variables and responses. Whiting (1968) was among the first to make use of the increase in the range of many variables through cross-cultural research. She greatly broadened the study of weaning ages, for instance, by observing weaning practices and their effects in a variety of countries. Another example concerns population density. In studying several societies in Africa ranging in density from 250 to 1400 people per square mile, Monroe and Monroe (1972) were able to determine that higher densities led to more responses indicative of withdrawal from others. Studying this relationship in only one country may have led to restriction in the range of the independent variable—people per square mile—with the result that the relationship would not be discovered. Similarly, when investigators compare studies from many different settings, more variation is included than can be the case if only one setting is used. Cross-cultural research allows for a better description and understanding of important variables (Triandis and Brislin, 1984).

Identification of Universals

Psychologists for the most part have neglected the problem of behavioral universals. Two reasons exist for this. First, though psychology was predominantly a European export and an American import, its constructs, methods, and findings have been taken as de facto universal. The second reason is more specific: The adherents of behaviorism and other psychological theories describe their findings as reflective of a natural science with "laws" that hold true for all human behavior, no matter in which culture or context it occurs (Lonner, 1980). Yet little evidence for the universality of these "laws" has been adduced.

In this study, we take the position that the question of psychological similarities across countries is both important to answer and open for empirical investigation. Studying universals, moreover, has the advantage that it tends to obviate the difficulties that exist in international research (e.g., translation problems), since most of these differences contribute to difference, not similarities, between groups.

Brislin (1983) held that research on universals will be one of comparative psychology's most important contributions to theory development. Solid evidence that a concept is universal or has a universal core meaning is the foundation for incorporation into a theoretical system that describes human functioning. Universality leads to testable hypotheses across cultures and later integration of findings into theories. Similarities, and establishing the generality of psychological findings, should be given first priority.

Lonner (1980) has developed a typology, or a possible taxonomy, of psychological universals that helps to organize the diverse literature. He approached this topic by first noting that, *biologically*, we are all of the same species; *socially*, the species is governed by generalized functional prerequisites; and *ecologically*, the species must adapt to a limited range of geographic and environmental conditions (ecosystems). These three bases for making comparisons across cultures converge into various patterns that form a finite number of culture types, thus allowing for the further comparison of individuals within the cultures along a fourth base—the *psychological*, which would assume an intraspecies commonality of processes.

Lonner identified seven types of universals that are pertinent to a psychological context, some of which are "strong and unequivocal," while others "defy empirical proof." They range from basic universals—such as all societies having some kind of language, laws and rules, and a common history—to supposed universals that either cannot be or have not yet been the topic of empirical research.

These seven types of psychologically oriented universals are relevant to our study since, as we shall see, the results show there are a significant number of items that are universally endorsed by the world's teenagers. And since the "universal items" (discussed in Chapter 4) come from six of ten OSIQ scales, we have evidence that there are issues or feelings with universal relevance among the world's teenagers. This fact, and the fact that teenagers, as we shall show, agreed on the valence or direction of their endorsements, has implications for a universal psychology of adolescence.

Difficulties of Comparative Studies

Cross-national researchers are faced with many problems. But there have emerged several useful approaches to dealing with the difficulties that exist. Following is a consideration of a few of the most common difficulties and how they have been approached, if not resolved, in this study.

Adjusting to Another Culture

When researchers work outside the familiar confines of their own society, there are some obvious initial difficulties (see Triandis and Brislin, 1984). There is a different language; there are different norms and customs; there are new interpersonal relations to which to become acclimated; and there may be distrust, intrusion, and long-term networks in which new researchers may not be welcome. One way to overcome these difficulties involves the use of collaborators. As noted earlier in this section (Brislin, 1983; Lambert, 1980), collaborative research with colleagues from other countries who have firsthand knowledge about the culture being studied is quite desirable. Local collaborators can help select representative samples to study, pave the way to accessing these samples, and facilitate subject cooperation. It is safe to say that our use of local collaborators for both translation and administration purposes mitigated the potential difficulty of adjusting to, and working in, a new culture.

Translation

In every comparative study researchers have to deal with the problem of translation between languages. Accuracy of translation, therefore, becomes a fundamental issue.

A common complaint is that certain concepts central to one culture may be difficult to phrase in the language of another. For example, the Japanese term *amae* describes what is thought to be a unique form of dependency, evident only among the Japanese (Doi, 1973). Though a concept may have different meanings in different languages or cultures, or this concept may appear to be missing in another culture, this simply should be a starting point for discussion and research (Triandis and Brislin, 1984). It may well be that what appears to be a fundamental difference is quite comprehensible when phrased in the appropriate constructs of another language.

To achieve the most appropriate translation, one or more of the four categories of translation (each having a different purpose) is utilized (Casagrande, 1954). Pragmatic translation refers to the translation of a message with an interest in the accuracy of the information meant to be conveyed; it is used most often in the translation of technical documents. Aesthetic-poetic translation, on the other hand, takes into account the affect, emotion, and feelings of an original-language version, as well as the aesthetic form and the information intended; it is most often used in the translation of literature. Ethnographic translation is used to explicate the cultural context of the source and second-language versions, and is sensitive to the specific way words (particularly slang terms) are used and fit into the culture. Finally, linguistic translation is concerned with achieving a translation of "equivalent meanings" in the second language. Though any one translation rarely fits into only one category, it was the linguistic type of translation that was closest to our purposes of conveying the meaning of the concepts used in the OSIQ from the first language to the second.

There are a variety of translation methods that can be employed in a multinational research project. Back-translation consists of preparing the material in one language, asking a bilingual to translate it into the target language, and then having a second bilingual independently translate the material back into the original language; items yielding discrepant responses can then be identified. The committee approach uses a group of bilinguals to translate from the source to the target language, creating a system of checks and balances. Pretest procedures call for field-testing the instrument before it is actually used for data collection to ensure that people will understand the material in the way it is meant (Brislin, 1980). In this study, we used a combination of approaches. A number of different translators in each language were consulted, both for initial translation purposes and for their responses to specific items. Some pretesting was carried out to check the accuracy of the translation. The greatest emphasis was put on back-translation. In addition, statistical techniques were employed to explore the viability of constructs as translated from English into other languages (see Chapter 3).

The Emic–Etic Distinction

Closely related to the different meaning problem in translation is the culture-specific meaning. This issue has to do with the distinction between the culture-common, or universal, dimensions of a concept (etic) and the culture-specific aspects of a concept (emic). The two terms are derived from the two systems of linguistics, phonemic (sounds employed within a single linguistic system) and phonetic (the more general or even universal aspects of language; Pike, 1966). A similar distinction is seen in formulations such as "inside" versus "outside" or "first-person" versus "third-person" descriptions (Geertz, 1984). The emic approach examines only one culture from an inside perspective. The etic approach examines many cultures, comparatively, from a perspective outside the culture. The emic approach seeks an understanding of a concept or construct as employed in that particular culture. The etic approach seeks to understand how a concept conceived by an outside researcher would fit many cultures (Berry, 1980).

While the emic approach is useful in obtaining culture-specific descriptions, the etic methodology facilitates making comparisons (Davidson, Jaccard, Triandis, Morales, and Diaz-Guerrero, 1976). In our case, we sought to discover images of the self across cultures using etic or external criteria. We also wished to discover emic content to the extent allowed by our methodology, however. We sought to discover emic, or local, images of the self. Even though we did not ask them to describe themselves in their own words, by their endorsements of certain items we obtained hints about unique aspects of teenagers' self-image in different nations.

In integrating the two, or utilizing a "combined emic–etic" approach (Davidson et al., 1976), we accomplished two goals of cross-national research. The first goal was documenting valid principles of behavior in any one culture by using constructs that the people themselves conceive as meaningful and important (emic analysis). The second goal was to make generalizations across cultures that take into account cross-national human behavior (etic analysis). This enabled us to gain access to both the local and universal aspects of the constructs that were used.

Testing across Cultures

The interpretation of test scores across cultures is an important issue. Trying to study constructs, compare meanings of test scores, and undertake item analyses across cultures has resulted in much debate, criticism, and controversy (Irvine and Carroll, 1980). Through the use of procedures described in the methodology chapter, item-scale analyses across cultures were generated. As Irvine and Carroll (1980) note, where there are no significant differences in the cross- and within-culture item correlations, one can be almost certain that the true score variances are similar in kind and amount. Such application of checks on data can greatly improve interpretation of these data.

Authenticity

A further criticism of cross-national research is that use of a single measuring device—for instance, a test to measure personality through self-report—may suffer from single-method bias. As Triandis and Brislin (1984) pointed out, this bias can occur in some cases through people flattering themselves in one culture and people tending to be self-deprecating in another. This bias can be dealt with by using as many different data-gathering techniques as possible.

Another way to gain control over this problem is to better understand whether the responses to the various questions are genuine or biased. Well-known methods are available for establishing reliability and validity. However, neither reliability nor validity guarantees authenticity. Parek and Rao (1980) make the point that while reliability and validity generally refer to the internal properties of the instrument itself, and whether the instrument really measures what it is supposed to measure, authenticity depends upon the respondent. Authenticity involves the investigator's ability to get unbiased, genuine, and accurate responses from the subject.

A number of cultural and various other factors contribute to the authenticity of responses, or lack thereof, as Parek and Rao (1980) noted. The four sets of factors affecting authenticity when the same standardized questionnaire is used in different cultures are investigator/collaborator-related factors, the test and its setting, respondent-related factors, and national or cultural factors. Examples are whether the collaborator was affiliated with a prestigious organization, since this might cause the respondent to take the questionnaire more seriously; the image the respondent has of the investigator; and the trust or alliance established between the investigator and the respondent, which is often based on similar socioeconomic status. One very salient issue is whether respondents from a certain culture tend to use a courtesy norm (giving answers that would be thought to please or satisfy the interviewer), or whether a game-playing norm (leading a stranger astray) existed. The point that Parek and Rao made is that care taken to control these factors favorably will improve the quality and the authenticity of the responses.

In our study, as much care as possible was taken with regard to these factors. Local collaborators, who would be expected to possess little bias, were used to administer the questionnaire. This helped to create a favorable image, a bond of trust with the respondents that their thoughts were important and valued by the researchers. These factors contributed to the authenticity of responses. The questionnaire was given anonymously in the students' own classroom. The students' assistance in the investigator's learning about teenagers' feelings and attitudes was sought. As a result, the students' motivation to answer honestly and accurately presumably was increased, contributing to authenticity. The collaborators' observations of the subjects themselves are discussed in greater detail in Chapter 3. There is no indication of bias due to previous experience. Finally, all these factors were closely monitored, as well as "the seven principles" of cross-cultural testing (Irvine and Caroll, 1980, pp. 196–197) being applied, both to lessen single-method bias and to deal with the cultural factors, thereby enhancing authenticity. It is clear, however, that authenticity-decreasing cultural factors, such as social desirability, cannot be *a priori* ruled out as contributory to results. The influence of these factors will be assessed when results are discussed.

Proving Universality

The guideline we used in this study was Triandis's (1978) statement that if one has evidence of cultural similarities from two or more cultures—and there is no available evidence contradicting the evidence of similarities—one is justified in hypothesizing that a process or relationship is universal. All our conclusions regarding universals were checked in multiple ways across all the nations studied.

Comparative Studies Reconsidered

As we have noted, research in comparative psychology is fraught with inherent difficulties, yet these difficulties are not insurmountable. This field of study, we believe, will soon reach a new level of maturity. Currently, there exists a limited view not only of the field itself but of the cross-national psychological diversity from which we attempt to draw our knowledge.

It is possible that within a generation our world view will have changed radically. It may well be that we will come to think in terms of a world culture, as we do now of a world economy. A world view of this nature would have great implications for intercultural research in psychology. It may be that the overriding issue in this field, certainly in the decades to come, will be how we view psychology and culture within the context of a world community.

Triandis and Brislin (1984) stated, "In an increasingly interdependent world the demands for cross-cultural training are growing." This training would focus on researchers' becoming more aware of and sensitive to cultural differences in order to better evaluate people from other cultural backgrounds in their studies. Triandis (1979) also pointed out that "a global society will require a much better understanding of universals." Our research is part of this quest to increase knowledge of cultural differences and similarities. The contribution of this study may be in providing a clear picture of cross-national differences and similarities in adolescents' view of themselves. This contribution rests on evidence that it is possible to understand the teenagers of other cultures. In particular, it rests on the possibility of being able to shed light on the self-image of adolescents from many different countries by using a standard instrument—an instrument that not only taps areas of universal concern to adolescents but also invites them in a non-threatening way to express what they really feel about themselves.

CHAPTER 3

Design and Procedure

Description of the Offer Self-Image Questionnaire • Description of Countries and Samples Studied • Data Analysis

An attempt to study adolescents raises questions about how anyone can know what adolescents are experiencing or feeling. Studying the human experience is *per se* difficult and complex. Studying adolescents seems particularly difficult since they are simultaneously as complex as, but different from, adults; yet it is adults who are trying to understand them.

To understand adolescents, adults often consult their own experience, rely on media imagery, or look to mental health professionals for guidance. However, a particular adult's experience of adolescence is always idiosyncratic and the memory of one's own adolescence is probably not totally veridical. The media are suffused with dramatic, often negative, imagery wherein adolescents are portrayed in stereotypical ways. The concepts that mental health professionals have of adolescents have been shown to be biased in a systematically negative way (Hartlage, Howard, and Ostrov, 1984; Offer, Ostrov, and Howard, 1981b).

The position we take is that to obtain sharable and useful knowledge about adolescence, data must be gathered in ways that are in the public domain and replicable. The contrasting data-gathering techniques are through use of anecdotes, impressions, and unique experiences with individual adolescents.

Our primary approach to research on adolescence has been to utilize self-report, structured questionnaires. The strengths of such an approach are that each teenage subject responds to the same set of stimuli. Items are written to cover important areas of functioning; by presenting all the items, the researcher can be assured that all of these areas are inquired about in some detail. In addition, responses are precoded and ready for analysis. Moreover, the use of a structured questionnaire allows for group testing. As a result, large samples can be investigated economically. In our experience, adolescents often feel more comfortable responding in an anonymous-structured format than they do talking with an adult interviewer. In addition, the researcher is not faced with the myriad problems involved in coding responses for analysis.

There are several weaknesses to such an approach, however. A major problem is that a teenager can provide responses only to the questions specifically posed. There is no opportunity for inquiring about aspects of his or her world that may be important to that particular teenager but were overlooked in the construction of the questionnaire. Furthermore, there is no opportunity for a more in-depth exploration of the answers that the teenagers do supply. In the final analysis, however, an investigator must choose a methodology. We have chosen an approach that allows for the collection of a large amount of standardized information that can be efficiently analyzed.

DESCRIPTION OF THE OFFER SELF-IMAGE QUESTIONNAIRE

Our approach to the measurement of self-image is to use the teenager's report of attitudes and feelings about his or her self in a number of important areas. To accomplish this, we utilized the Offer Self-Image Questionnaire (OSIQ). The OSIQ is a self-descriptive personality test that assesses the adjustment of teenage boys and girls between the ages of 13 and 19. It comprises 130 items concerning teenagers' feelings about their psychological world. (For the background of the OSIQ, its reliability, validity, and standard scoring methodology, see Offer, Ostrov, and Howard, 1981a, 1982, 1984.)

The OSIQ is designed for group administration. It was devised so that it combines simplicity in responding for subjects, with ease of computer scoring for investigators. Subjects are asked to read the first page of the test booklet and provide the requested personal information (e.g., age). Alternatively, the examiner may choose to read the instructions and examples aloud, or have the subjects read them and ask questions. There is no time limit; each subject is to proceed at his or her own pace. Approximately 40 minutes are ordinarily required for completion. The great majority of subjects tested thus far have reacted positively to the experience.

The task presented to the subjects is to indicate how well each item describes them. A verbal description for each of the six response alternatives is provided at the top of each page of the test booklet. The subjects respond by circling a number (1 through 6) that is printed next to each item number on the answer sheet. The six response alternatives are as follows:

1. Describes me very well.
2. Describes me well.
3. Describes me fairly well.
4. Does not quite describe me.
5. Does not really describe me.
6. Does not describe me at all.

Since 1962 the OSIQ has been administered to over 400 samples of adolescents. It has been administered to over 30,000 teenagers in the United States alone. Samples include younger and older, normal, delinquent, psychiatrically disturbed, physically ill, urban, suburban, and rural boys and girls. The OSIQ has also been translated into 22 languages.

The OSIQ is based on two assumptions. First, it is necessary to evaluate the functioning of a person in multiple areas, since people can master one aspect of their world while failing to adjust in another. Second, the psychological sensitivity of adolescents is sufficiently acute to allow us to rely on their responses to the items in the questionnaire. Empirical work with the OSIQ has supported both of these assumptions (Offer et al., 1981a, 1984).

The 130 items of the OSIQ are organized into 11 scales. These in turn are conceptualized in terms of five "selves," as described below.

Psychological Self (PS)

The Psychological Self comprises the adolescents' concerns, feelings, wishes, and fantasies. The scales that constitute this self deal with the teenagers' sense of control over impulses, the emotions, and conceptions of their bodies. The three relevant OSIQ scales follow.

PS-1: Impulse Control. This scale measures the extent to which the ego apparatus of the adolescents is strong enough to cope with various pressures that exist in their internal and external environments.

Positive item—Even under pressure, I manage to remain calm.
Negative item—I get violent if I don't get my way.

PS-2: Emotional Tone. This scale measures the degree of affective harmony within the psychic structure; it measures the valence of the dolescents' moods as well as the extent to which there is fluctuation in emotions.

Positive item—I enjoy life.
Negative item—I am so very anxious.

PS-3: Body Image. This scale indicates the extent to which the adolescents feel positive or feel awkward about their bodies.

Positive item—I am proud of my body.
Negative item—I frequently feel ugly and unattractive.

Social Self (SS)

Adolescents are often described in terms of the friends they have, the company they keep, and the values they hold. In the Social Self, adolescents' perception of their interpersonal relationships, their moral attitudes, and their vocational and educational goals are assessed. The three relevant OSIQ scales in this area follow.

SS-1: Social Relationships. This scale assesses peer relationships and friendship patterns.

Positive item—Being together with other people gives me a good feeling.
Negative item—I prefer being alone to being with kids my age.

SS-2: Morals. This scale measures the extent to which the conscience or superego has developed.

Positive item—I would not hurt someone just for the "heck of it."
Negative item—Telling the truth means nothing to me.

SS-3: Vocational and Educational Goals. One of the specific tasks of the adolescent is learning and planning for a vocational future. This scale measures how well the teenager is faring in accomplishing this task.

Positive item—A job well done gives me pleasure.
Negative item—I feel that working is too much responsibility for me.

Sexual Self (S×S)

This aspect of the self concerns an area of functioning that is of vital concern in adolescence: the integration of emerging sexual drives into psychosocial life. With respect to this area, we ask adolescents how they feel about their sexual experiences and behavior. The following scale is used.

S×S: *Sexual Attitudes.* This scale concerns itself with the adolescent's feelings, attitudes, and behaviors toward sexual matters.

Positive item—Sexual experiences give me pleasure.
Negative item—Thinking or talking about sex frightens me.

Familial Self (FS)

The feelings and attitudes teenagers have toward their families are crucial for their overall psychological health. Barring extreme circumstances, the family will contribute more to the development of adolescents than will any other psychosocial influence. The following scale is used.

FS: *Family Relationships.* This scale is concerned with how the adolescents feel about their parents and the kind of relationships they have with them. It assesses the emotional atmosphere of the home.

Positive item—I can count on my parents most of the time.
Negative item—I try to stay away from home most of the time.

Coping Self (CS)

The scales constituting this aspect of the self measure the psychiatric symptoms the adolescents say they have, if any; they also allow the adolescents to describe how they cope with the world. The three relevant OSIQ scales follow.

CS-1: *Mastery of the External World.* This scale assesses how well an adolescent adapts to the immediate environment.

Positive item—When I decide to do something, I do it.
Negative item—I feel that I have no talent whatsoever.

CS-2: Psychopathology. This scale identifies overt psychopathology.

> Positive item—No one can harm me just by not liking me.
> Negative item—I am confused most of the time.

CS-3: Superior Adjustment. This scale measures how the adolescents feel about their ability to cope and could also be defined as a measure of ego strength.

> Positive item—Dealing with new intellectual subjects is a challenge for me.
> Negative item—If I would be separated from all people I know, I feel that I would not be able to make a go of it.

Aside from being highly structured and objectively scored, the OSIQ represents an attempt to learn about people through asking them what they believe and how they feel. To this extent the OSIQ represents an attempt to understand the phenomenal world of the subject. Yet, though the OSIQ allows adolescents to describe themselves from their own point of view, it nevertheless could be thought of as using an etic methodology. (An etic approach, as described earlier on pp. 30–31, refers to use of a transcultural standard to understand phenomena in a particular culture. It contrasts with an emic approach, also described on pp. 30–31, which refers to attempting to understand phenomena in a particular culture from the point of view of persons in that culture, not from some external, "objective" standard.) The reason the OSIQ could be said to be etic is that it contains *a priori* scales that are made up, in a predesignated way, of certain items. The questionnaire does not allow for dimensions or components of dimensions that may be idiosyncratic or unique to a particular culture. It does not allow for the possibility that an item may represent one aspect of self for one culture and a different aspect of self for a different culture. The OSIQ is etic in that in effect it sets in advance which dimensions are of interest. One correction was that if a particular item showed a relationship to a scale in one country and a different relationship in other countries, then that item was eliminated from our study. A contrasting methodology would have allowed adolescents to state what is salient to them and would have inquired about that. There would have been an emphasis on identifying why that item behaved uniquely in the particular culture.

The disadvantage of using an etic method was that we did not gather information about all the dimensions of functioning important in particular cultures; we did not obtain data about unique associations of items within particular dimensions in specific cultures.

The advantage of our methodology, however, was that we maximized the opportunity to compare adolescents across countries along given dimensions. The OSIQ could be viewed as providing an opportunity for adolescents to agree on certain aspects of self-experience. The OSIQ by no means ensured that universal affirmation would be found, however. There was room for a great deal of disagreement in each dimension. While using a more purely emic approach would have rendered finding universals less likely, using the OSIQ by no means guaranteed generating areas of universal agreement across adolescents.

In analyzing results, we saw no evidence that much information was lost in using an etic method. On the contrary, most adolescents seem to easily understand common dimensions such as impulse control, body image, family relationships, and coping. It was a rare exception that an item uniquely loaded on a particular dimension for a certain culture. In those instances when loadings were not appropriate, a mistranslation usually seemed responsible—not a unique association of a particular idea or attitude with a dimension of adolescent experience for a particular culture.

It should be emphasized that the methodology used in this book did not ensure the direction of any universal agreement found. The instrument used allowed for as much agreement about negative aspects of experience as about positive aspects of experience. The fact that the areas of agreement reflect positive attitudes and feelings is a testimony to the enthusiasm and confidence of youth.

Sampling and Procedure

Since the publication of the OSIQ, we have received many requests from investigators throughout the world for copies of the questionnaire. In 1982 we wrote to investigators in other countries, who had asked to use the OSIQ, to request their cooperation in a multinational study of adolescent self-image.

Sixteen investigators from ten different countries provided the data that we used in this book. Each of these investigators did his or her own data collection in the native language of each country. Where necessary, the investigator translated the OSIQ items into the appropriate language. In all cases the raw data were sent to us and analyzed at our own computer facility. Investigators whose countries are not repre-

sented in this book included persons who could not get permission
from relevant authorities to collect the required data. Others did not
have access to appropriate samples (see Chapter 1). Table 1 shows the
composition of our final sample.

DESCRIPTION OF COUNTRIES AND SAMPLES STUDIED

Before describing the specific methods we used in this study, it is
important to give an overview of the ten countries in which the study
took place from an economic, demographic, and educational perspective, since these factors obviously affect adolescents' growing up in
these countries. In describing these countries, we restricted ourselves
to variables that were available across all or most of the countries and at
the same time communicate the "flavor" of each country. We will also
describe the samples from the ten countries focusing on their socioeconomic characteristics and how they were selected.

Tables 2 and 3 display a variety of characteristics of the ten countries in our sample (some data were not available for some countries).
With regard to demography, we report total population and population
density (people per square mile of land). Among economic variables we
report gross national product (GNP), per capita income, unemployment
rate, and quality of life index (based on literacy, life expectancy, and
infant mortality). Percent of 14- to 18-year-olds in the population, per

TABLE 1. Number of Adolescents Participating in the Multinational Study[a]

	Younger males	Older males	Younger females	Older females
Australia	98	96	136	149
Bangladesh	99	91	110	92
Hungary	278	287	291	301
Israel	82	191	101	206
Italy	358	276	335	281
Japan[b]	—	202	—	209
Taiwan	55	128	45	135
Turkey	99	133	89	129
United States	123	123	123	122
West Germany	78	88	93	106
Total	1,270	1,615	1,323	1,730

[a] Grand total of adolescents who participated in the multinational study: $N = 5,938$.
[b] The sample of younger males and females from Japan was too small for inclusion.

TABLE 2. Population Characteristics of the Ten Countries

	Population[a]	People per square mile[b]	GNP[c]	Per capita income[d]	Unemployment rate[e]	Quality of life index[f]
Australia	16	5	142.2	9,820	5.8	96
Bangladesh	100	1,791	11.2	120	—	36
Hungary	10	297	45.0	4,180	—	91
Israel	4	512	17.4	4,500	4.9	92
Italy	57	490	368.9	6,480	8.4	95
Japan	120	835	1,152.9	9,890	2.2	98
Taiwan	19	1,530	50.6	2,579	1.3	88
Turkey	50	167	66.1	1,460	1.5	62
West Germany	61	640	827.8	13,590	5.5	94
United States	237	65	2,582.5	11,360	9.6	96

[a] Estimated population in 1984 in millions (UNESCO, 1984).
[b] Estimated for 1984 (UNESCO, 1984).
[c] GNP = Gross National Product in billions of U.S. dollars (*1980 World Book Atlas*; Kurian, 1984).
[d] Per capita income is given in U.S. dollars (*1980 International Office Statistics*; Kurian, 1984).
[e] Percent of persons of working age who are unemployed (*1980 International Labor Office Statistics*; Kurian, 1984).
[f] A composite index calculated by averaging three indices—life expectancy, infant mortality, and literacy—covering the period 1981. Each index is rated on a scale from 1 to 100 and given equal weight in the averaging (*Overseas Development Council*; Kurian, 1984).

capita educational expenditure, percent of school-aged children actually enrolled in school, percent of 15- to 19-year-olds in the labor force, and marriage rates for 15- to 19-year-olds are of importance for understanding adolescents' experience.

First, let us present an overview of the factors presented in Tables 2 and 3, and their impact on each country. This is, obviously, not an all-inclusive description of each country. It is a bird's-eye view in which we give the reader an understanding about the kind of country in which the adolescent is growing up. We shall also describe each country's sample.

Australia

Australia is the sixth largest country in the world. Its relatively small population is associated with its having one of the lowest population densities in the world: only five people per square mile. But most Australians experience urban living, not vast open areas, since almost

TABLE 3. Adolescent Characteristics of the Ten Countries

	Percent 14–18[a]	Education expenditure per capita[b]	Percent secondary school-aged children who are actually enrolled[c]	Percent of 15- to 19-year-olds in labor force[d]		Marriage rate among 15- to 19-year-olds[e]	
				Males	Females	Males	Females
Australia	8.4	505	86	48	48	2	7
Bangladesh	10.8	2	15	72	19	8	76
Hungary	6.5	167	40	41	43	2	14
Israel	8.7	389	71	35	34	1	8
Italy	7.8	259	73	44	36	1	7
Japan	7.4	508	91	33	32	0	1
Taiwan	8.8	66	—	—	—	—	—
Turkey	10.8	48	37	56	45	8	12
West Germany	8.1	566	90	57	57	0	4
United States	7.7	676	96	39	32	3	9

[a] Based on 1985 projection of statistics for 1982, determined by estimating the percent of population aged 15–19 from the percent of population aged 15–24, using the projected population aged 15–19 and the projected population aged 20–24, and then multiplying that percentage by the total population and comparing the result to the projected population aged 15–19, and finally adjusting for a 1-year shift downward of the age group (United Nations, 1985).

[b] Educational expenditures per capita for 1980 given in U.S. dollars (Kurian, 1984).

[c] From UNESCO sources for the period covering 1979–1980. Secondary-school age for these nine countries ranges from 10–14 for the youngest to 16–18 for the oldest (Kurian, 1984).

[d] 1985 projection of trends for 1950–1970, as determined by the International Labor Organization. Economically active persons are defined as those working for pay or profit at any time during a specified period or who are seeking such work; included are unpaid family work, any kind of self-employment, and production of primary products such as foodstuffs, for own consumption, and does not need to be full time (United Nations, 1985).

[e] Rate per 100; data collected between 1974 and 1981 (United Nations, 1985).

nine out of ten Australians live in the urban centers along the south-west and southeast coasts.

Australia is a nation of immigrants. It ranks third in volume of immigration, behind only the United States and Canada. The dominant religion of Australians is Christian, with the remainder being Jews, Muslims, Buddhists, and Confucians. The life-style, in the coastal urban areas, largely reflects that of Western Europe.

With a varied economic base of agriculture, rural industries, mining, manufacturing, and services (the last of which accounts for almost three-fourths of its total employment), Australia's per capita income is among the highest in the world. Its quality of life, as measured by the United Nations, is among the best in the world.

There are about 1.3 million teenagers aged 14 to 18 in Australia, representing about 8% of the population. School attendance is mandatory from age 6 to 15 in all but one state, where it is mandatory to age 16. Most Australian high schools are modern, coeducational, and multipurpose, offering a curriculum similar to British and North American schools. Australia spends $505 (U.S.) per capita on education, ranking it fourth on this variable among the countries studied. Of teenagers 12 to 15 years of age, 86% are enrolled in secondary schools. Forty-eight percent of Australian teenagers 15 to 19 years of age are in the labor force.

Australia's political institutions follow the British democratic tradition, with an elected Parliament. The Parliament is the legislative branch of government, consisting of the House of Representatives and the Senate. Though the king or queen of Great Britain is the sovereign ruler, the executive cabinet, elected by the Parliament, is the major policy-making agency of the government and is presided over by the prime minister. There are four main political parties represented in the Australian Parliament, all of which support the maintenance of parliamentary democracy.

The Australian Sample was collected by Dr. P. W. Musgrave, professor of education at Monash University. The 479 Australian adolescents were from a state high school in a suburb of Melbourne, the second largest city (population of 2.8 million) in the country. The suburb consists primarily of "middle Australia," or lower-middle- and upper-working-class people. The OSIQ was introduced as part of a research project that was being conducted at Monash University, and was administered (in English) to all of the students present on the day of testing. The teenagers in this sample ranged in age from 13 to 18. They were cooperative and completed the questionnaire with very few questions and no complaints.

Bangladesh

With 1,791 people per square mile, Bangladesh has the highest population density of any nation in the world. The dominant religion in Bangladesh is Islam, with Hinduism contributing a small percentage.

Bangladesh is the third poorest country in the world and has one of the lowest per capita incomes. The country is considered one of the least developed countries in the world and, in particular, one of the countries most adversely affected by unrestricted population growth and natural disaster. Against a background of poverty, the cost of living in the capital city of Dacca is comparable to that in Washington, D.C. Not surprisingly, the quality of life index for Bangladesh is lowest among the countries studied. Despite these discouraging facts, Bangladesh ranks fourth in the world in rice production. There has been a recent attempt to encourage industrialization.

Education is compulsory in Bangladesh through age 10. The educational system consists of primary, secondary, and vocational schools, with higher education for the relatively few. Eleven million persons, 11% of the total population, are between the ages of 14 and 18. Fifteen percent of those of secondary-school age actually are enrolled in secondary school. Educational expenditures amount to $2 (U.S.) per capita or 1.7% of the gross national product. Seventy-two percent of males and 19% of females ages 15 to 19 were in the labor force in 1985. of 15- to 19-year-olds, 8% of boys are married, while 76% of Bengali girls are married—a rate more than five times higher than that of the next highest rate in this category among the ten countries studied.

Though Bangladesh came under military rule in December of 1983, martial law was lifted in December of 1986 when General Erhsad was elected president of Bangladesh.

The Bangladesh Sample was collected by Muhammad Nazmul Haq of Mymensing Teachers' Training College in Mymensing. This sample comprises 392 students, ranging in age from 13 to 18, from two boys' secondary schools, two girls' secondary schools, and one coeducational college—all located in the urban areas of Dacca and the neighboring district of Tangail. The large majority of these teenagers were from a middle- to upper-middle-class background, which was a determining factor in selecting these particular schools and students. Since these teenagers had never participated in a self-evaluative study, completing the Bengali-language version of the OSIQ was a completely new experience. However, complete explanations and instructions were given (based on the OSIQ manual), and the students adjusted well and completed the questionnaire with little difficulty. They were enthusiastic about the study, and many asked for their individual results.

Hungary

One of the oldest nations in Europe, Hungary has only recently been transformed from an agrarian to an industrial economy. It has a steadily increasing gross national product and per capita income. It is ranked second in the world in percentage of labor force in industry, sixth in food production, and seventh in land under cultivation. Hungary also ranks sixth in number of physicians and first in number of professional theatrical companies and amateur troupes, while maintaining one of the lowest unemployment rates of any country. At the same time, Hungary ranks first in suicide rate among its inhabitants (adolescents included). The suicide rate per 100,000 inhabitants is 43.1; by comparison, the suicide rate in the United States is 13.3 per 100,000.

Education is free and compulsory in Hungary from age 6 to 14. Budapest, a modern capital city with 2 million people, is the center of Hungarian intellectual life, with 85% of the country's research workers and scholars located there. One of every four high school students, and almost half of Hungary's university students, study in Budapest.

The percentage of 14- to 18-year-olds among the Hungarian population—6.5%—is relatively low. Of the two-thirds of a million teenagers of secondary school age, 40% are still attending school. Hungary spends $167 (U.S.) per capita on education, a relatively low amount. Forty-two percent of Hungarian adolescents 15 to 19 years of age were in the labor force in 1985. Two percent of 15- to 19-year-old males and 14% of 15- to 19-year-old females are married.

Hungary is a People's Republic, with its legislative power vested in the unicameral National Assembly (parliament). Its 352 members are elected for four-year terms. The supreme body of state power is the 21-member Presidential Council elected by the National Assembly. The only political party of the country is the Communist Hungarian Socialist Workers' Party.

The Hungarian Sample was collected by Dr. Mária Kertész, specialist for pediatrics and adolescent medicine in Budapest. Most adolescents from the Hungarian sample were enrolled in four public high schools in Budapest. Two schools were academic high schools whose students came from nearby districts. The other schools were technical secondary high schools that drew their students from all districts of Budapest and outskirts as well as nearby rural areas. Some of the students lived in dormitories in the capital. Some of the younger adolescents were recruited from primary schools from the same districts. To make the sample more representative, students from different summer camps were also included. This student group came from practically all parts of the country. The Hungarian version of the OSIQ was completed by 565 boys and 592 girls between the ages of 13 and 19.

Permission to participate was sought and granted through the Board of Education of the schools. Generally, classrooms were used to obtain access to students. The subjects, after being provided information about the benefits of the test, were highly cooperative. The OSIQ was administered in Hungarian. It was welcomed by the vast majority of the Hungarian adolescents as a way to gain new self-knowledge. There were some students who voluntarily visited the outpatient clinic a few days after they had filled out the OSIQ for consultations on particular items. This also indicated that interest in self-knowledge was initiated by the OSIQ.

Israel

In Israel, a cosmopolitan nation with ancient roots, almost 90% of the 4 million people are urban dwellers. Jews, mostly immigrants since 1948, currently make up 83% of the total population. Other religions represented are Christian, Moslem, and Bahai.

Though lacking in natural resources, extensive arable land, and commercial ties with nearby countries, Israel has become an industrial state and increased its GNP by 2000% since 1950. Its per capita income is now $4,500, ranking it among the leading countries in the world.

A little over one-third of Israel's workers are in service industries; tourism is a $1 billion-a-year industry. Manufacturing employs 27% and agriculture 6% of workers. Women make up over one-third of the labor force, while 5% of the labor force are unemployed. Israel has the highest soldier–civilian ratio of the countries studied here. Three-year service for men (18 to 29) and two-year service for single women (18 to 25) is compulsory in the Israel Defense Forces, which is allocated 24% of the national budget.

Israel is an education-oriented society; one in every three Israelis is a student in some kind of educational program. Education is free and compulsory for all children aged 5 to 16. Israel expends 8.3% of its GNP, or $389 per capita, on education. Seventy-one percent of teenagers aged 14 to 17 are enrolled in secondary schools. Thirty-five percent of Israeli teenagers were in the labor force as of 1985. The marriage rate among Israeli teenagers is relatively low—1% for males and 8% for females.

Israeli is a parliamentary democracy. It has general elections to select members to its Parliament (Knesset). There are many parties that form coalitions. A coalition that can muster a simple majority in the Knesset selects the prime minister, who, in turn, selects his cabinet.

The Israeli Sample was provided from studies conducted by Dr. Rachel Seginer, of the University of Haifa, and Dr. Amiram Raviv, of Tel Aviv University. In each case the OSIQ was administered in Hebrew. The total sample included 580 Israeli-Jewish adolescents with ages ranging from 14 to 18. Dr. Seginer's subjects came from a comprehensive school just outside of Haifa. Three major programs are offered by the school—academic matriculation, vocational matriculation, and vocational without matriculation. The school is especially known for its vocational matriculation program, particularly in high-technology areas. The community consists mostly of middle-class families and some new immigrants. Thirty-one percent of the students' parents were born in Israel, 44% in Europe and the Americas, and 20% in Middle Eastern or North African countries. Most of the parents had an education that went beyond high school. Freshmen and seniors in the academic and vocational matriculation programs were tested. Psychology and education majors from the University of Haifa served as research assistants, administering the OSIQ to groups during regular class periods. Extensive preparation preceded administration of the OSIQ—securing permission, meeting with homeroom teachers, and getting feedback from the potential subjects. On the whole, the students were responsive and cooperative in their participation.

Dr. Raviv's subjects were from two comprehensive high schools in urban Tel Aviv and the junior and senior high schools of a nearby suburb, Kiryat Ono. The socioeconomic background of these students was middle to upper middle class. Nearly 90% of these adolescents go on to pursue a higher education of some kind. All of the students present in the selected (9th through 11th grades) classrooms were tested using the Hebrew version of the OSIQ, having been told that the investigators wanted to know how the subjects think and feel about themselves and various issues concerning teenagers. They were told they would be taking part in an "international research study." The participants took the task seriously and seemed to enjoy taking the OSIQ.

Italy

Tracing its roots to the ancient Roman empire, Italy is today in the vanguard of the modern, technologically advanced nations of Europe. Italy is the 13th most populous nation in the world, and 5th in our study. Roman Catholicism is the predominant religion of Italians.

Italy is poorly endowed in natural resources yet ranks fourth in industrial power among the European nations. Its GNP is seventh highest in the world. Per capita income is $6,480. At the same time, the unemployment rate in Italy is relatively high—8.4%.

Free public education is mandatory in Italy from age 6 to 14. The Ministry of Education in Rome hires teachers and establishes curricula and syllabi. After middle school, students who decide to continue their education can choose among many different types of secondary schools, including lyceums (classical, scientific, and linguistic), teacher training schools, technical institutes, vocational training institutes, and schools for education in the arts. After middle school, 90% of the students go on to a higher degree, 73% go to secondary schools, and 30% go on to professional schools. Despite all this emphasis on education, Italy ranks only 25th in the world in educational expenditures per capita; $259 per capita is spent on education. The 14-to-18 age group make up 7.8% of the total population, with approximately 70% of them living in urban areas. Many Italian youths aged 15 to 19 work: 60% of boys and 40% of girls aged 15 to 19 were in the labor force in 1985. Relatively few Italian teenagers aged 15 to 19 marry: 1% of the boys and 7% of the girls.

The Italian Republic is governed by a two-house parliament (Senate and Chamber of Deputies), which elects a president for a term of seven years. The president nominates the premier, who recommends members of the cabinet. There are nine political parties holding seats in the chamber of deputies, with the Christian Democratic Party and the Communist Party the two leading parties.

The Italian Sample (1250 teenagers) was collected by Dr. Enrico de Vito of the Center for Clinical Psychology in Milan. The students ranged in age from 14 to 18 and were attending two secondary schools in the Milan area. One school is a technical-commercial institute of Sesto San Giovanni (a densely populated industrial town contiguous with Milan) offering training for various technical professions. A relatively small percentage of these students will pursue higher education. The teenagers were generally from lower-middle-class backgrounds. The other school is a scientific lyceum of Milan that offers university programs. The students primarily were from a middle- or upper-middle-class background. In each school, the OSIQ was administered in Italian as part of a research program on normality and vulnerability factors in adolescence being conducted by the Center for Clinical Psychology. The questionnaires were administered by teachers after briefing by the investigator. All of the students present in the selected classroom were tested, having been told that the questionnaire was a way to find out how they think and feel about themselves. The students completed the OSIQ with interest and without difficulty.

Japan

The fourth oldest nation in the world, Japan is today the seventh most populous. It is expected to reach a stationary population around 2045. In life expectancy, Japanese men and women are among the highest ranked in the world, along with Iceland. Buddhism was introduced into Japan from India through China in 538 A.D. and is today the major religion of the country, with Shintoism next.

It has been predicted that Japan will be the number one economic power in the world by the year 2000. Its GNP ($1.5 trillion) is second only to the United States and the Soviet Union. Per capita income is $9,890. Japan is the world's leading producer of ships, automobiles, television sets, and radios, as well as being the world's leading fishing nation. The quality of life index for Japan was highest among the nations studied here.

Japan's teenagers represent 7.4% of the total population, one of the lowest ratios of the countries studied. For all children aged 6 to 15, public education in Japan is free and compulsory. Almost three-fourths of all pupils in kindergarten, one-fourth in upper secondary schools, and three-fourths in higher education are enrolled in private schools. Japan also has "cram" schools, called juku, where students go to get additional help, particularly in becoming prepared for higher education. Though this often creates great pressure on the students, Japan now ranks second in scientific and engineering manpower. Ninety-one percent of teenagers aged 12 through 17 are enrolled in secondary schools. About one-third of Japanese teenagers aged 15 to 19 were in the labor force in 1985. The marriage rate among Japanese teenagers was the lowest of all the countries studied here (for which data were available): Less than 1% of Japanese boys and girls aged 15 through 19 are married.

The Japanese Republic is governed by an elected house of representatives (the Diet). The Diet selects a prime minister, who presides over the cabinet, which holds the executive power of the government. The emperor is the symbol of the state, though he holds no powers. There are currently six political parties in Japan, with the Liberal Democratic Party holding the majority of seats in the Diet, and the Socialist Party second.

The Japanese Sample was collected, under the direction of Dr. Shiroe Miura, professor of psychiatry at Tokyo Medical College, by Dr.

Sadao Ohshima, professor of sociology and psychology at the University of Meiji-Gakuin, and by Yukuhiko Miyoshi, P.S.W., teacher of high school at Katoh-Gakuen High School. The sample was composed of 411 16- to 18-year-old boys and girls from a private high school in Numazu City. These students were primarily from an upper-middle-class background. They completed the Japanese language version of the OSIQ diligently and asked no questions of the examiners.

Taiwan

Formerly known as Formosa, the island of Taiwan is today a stronghold of traditional Chinese culture. Taiwan, officially known as the Republic of China, has a relatively high population density (1,530 people per square mile). It is primarily a Buddhist country, although Taoism, Christianity, and Islam are also represented.

Since World War II, Taiwan has been the most prosperous province in Chinese history, having transformed its agrarian economy into an industrial one. It is now the 42nd richest country in the world, and it has overtaken mainland China and some developed nations in many areas of trade and manufacturing. It has an extremely low unemployment rate (1.3%). It has a current per capita income of $2,579; it is anticipated that by the 1990s this will reach $6,000. At that time Taiwan will become a fully developed country. Leading industries include electronics, petroleum, construction, and textiles.

Teenagers represent 8.8% of the total population of Taiwan. Education is free for all for nine years, from age 6 through 15. More than one-fourth of the population is in school, making a total of over 5 million students. Ninety-seven percent of the primary school graduates in 1981 went on to junior high, which has college prep and vocational courses.

Though Taiwan is nominally a republic with power resting in the hands of the people, martial law has been in effect since 1949. The president is head of the one-party system.

The Taiwanese Sample was collected by Sara Turner, a visiting professor from Humboldt State University in California. After contacts were made in a number of schools, a sample of 363 teenagers was selected from public schools in the modern city of Taichung, which has a population of over 500,000. Students from grades 9 through 12 were randomly selected by identification numbers and were administered the Chinese (Cantonese)-language version of the OSIQ. The subjects were mostly from middle-class families. They were very cooperative throughout the testing and maintained a pleasant mood.

Turkey

With a history going back more than 2,600 years, Turkey is the 19th most populous country in the world, with 50 million people concentrated in the west and along the coastal areas of the Mediterranean and Aegean seas. It has one of the highest annual population growth rates we studied. Ninety-nine percent of the population is Moslem, while Christian and Jewish minorities are also present.

Since 1980, when inflation began to erode gains in manufacturing, mining, and employment, Turkey placed its economic priorities on exports to strengthen its balance of payments. This resulted in a doubling of the export volume and an increase of 5.9% in its gross national product.

Today Turkey is the 28th largest economy in the world. It is strongest in the agricultural sector, ranking fifth in sheep, ninth in barley production, eighth in cotton fiber production, and seventh in wheat production. The per capita income of Turkey is relatively low (second lowest of the countries studied here). The quality of life index for Turkey is second lowest of the ten countries. For these reasons, Turkey is still considered to be an underdeveloped country.

Education in Turkey is mandatory from 6 to 12 years of age. The adolescent population (14 through 18) makes up 10.8% of the total population, with 54% living in urban areas. Thirty-seven percent of all 11- to 16-year-olds are enrolled in secondary schools, the second lowest proportion of the countries studied. Many older Turkish teenagers work, with 56% of the boys and 45% of the girls aged 15 through 19 in the labor force in 1985. Marriage rates among teenagers are somewhat higher than they are for most industrialized countries: 8% of 15- to 19-year-old boys and 12% of 15- to 19-year-old girls were married.

Since the 1960s a series of military and coalition governments have ruled Turkey. In 1980 the National Security Council, headed by a prime minister, was established. In 1983 the Motherland Party won over half the seats in the Grand National Assembly, with the Populist Party winning over a quarter of the seats.

The Turkish Sample was collected by Dr. Banu İnanc, assistant professor of psychology at Çukurova University. The subjects were from a private and a public school in Adana, a city of over 1 million people located near the southeastern coast of the country. The 450 students in this sample were mostly from urban upper-middle-class families and were considered above-average students, with ages ranging from 13 to 18. Approximately 10% of the sample were living in dormitories. The Turkish version of the OSIQ was administered in those classes that did not have any makeup lectures or examinations and therefore had the time to give one class period to the study. Subjects took the questionnaire seriously and had an interest in its purpose and how it would be evaluated.

United States

The 16th oldest nation and the 4th most populous, the United States has three-fourths of its population living in urban areas. Immigrants from every continent have made the United States one of the most ethnically diverse nations in the world. Christianity is the most prominent religion, with almost all other major religions being practiced as well.

With just 5% of the world's population and 6% of the land surface, the United States produces one-fourth of the gross global product. It is the world's leading industrial nation and dominates in the agricultural sector also. Its GNP was by far the largest of the nations studied here—per capita income is $11,360. The U.S. quality of life index is tied for second highest with Australia among the ten countries studied. Nevertheless, the U.S. employment rate is 9.6%—the highest among the ten nations—while 15% of the population lives below the poverty level. U.S. teenagers make up 7.7% of the total population, a relatively low percent. The U.S. educational system has been criticized for falling short of the excellence that it could attain given its resources, but it is still close to the top in many educational areas: first in graduate student population, foreign students in national universities, postsecondary enrollment, and number of university professors. With a mandatory school attendance from age 6 to 16, the United States ranks second in the world to the Soviet Union in secondary-school enrollment ratio, with 96% of secondary-school-aged children still in school. The $676 per capita spent by the United States on education was the highest of the nations studied. About 35% of U.S. teenagers 15 through 19 years old were in the labor force in 1985. The marriage rate for 15- to 19-year-olds is relatively high, being about 3% of boys and 9% of girls.

The United States follows the British tradition of democratic government. An elected president holds executive powers for a four-year term. Legislative power resides in a bicameral Congress whose members are elected periodically.

The United States Sample is taken from seven studies conducted in the 1980s on American teenagers. The total sample consists of 491 subjects, 13 to 18 years old. Drs. Offer, Ostrov, and Howard collected data on 155 students from a public high school in an affluent suburb of Chicago, Illinois. These teenagers were from middle- to upper-middle-class families. Dr. Anne Petersen of the Pennsylvania State University provided data on 56 students from another suburb of Chicago. They were randomly drawn as part of a larger investigation of biopsycho-social development during adolescence. These subjects were from lower-middle- to upper-middle-class backgrounds. Dr. Henry K. Watanabe of the United States Army collected data on the children of 132 army officers and recruits. Dr. David Hall of Johns Hopkins University provided data on 56 subjects from an inner-city area of Baltimore, Maryland. Dr. Wen Shing Tseng of the University of Hawaii Medical School collected data on 36 teenagers who volunteered for a normal family interaction study; these subjects were from middle- and upper-middle-class backgrounds and had ethnic backgrounds that included American or European, Japanese, Chinese, and Hawaiian ancestries. Marjorie Steinfeld provided data on 36 students from a private school in New York City. Lastly, Emily Ets-Hokin collected data on 20 students from a suburban high school near Chicago; these subjects were from a middle-class background and were a control group for her study of learning-disabled adolescents. For each American subsample, the original pool of subjects studied was much larger. We sampled from each in order to ensure that all individual data sets contained an equal number of younger and older boys and girls—so that each contributed in the same proportion to each of the four age-gender groups.

West Germany

The 12th most populous nation in the world, West Germany has a density of a little above 640 people per square mile. Ninety-four percent of the population are Christian (49% Protestant and 45% Catholic). Germany was divided into two separate nations following World War II. West Germany is one of Europe's strongest industrial powers as well as the world's second most important trading nation after the United States. Its primary products are iron, steel, coal, machinery, ships, and other vehicles. West Germany's gross national product is the fourth highest in the world, and its per capita income, $13,590, is highest among the nations studied here.

Adolescents constitute 8.1% of the West German population. The West German educational system is based on mandatory attendance from 6 to 16, and includes primary, postsecondary, secondary modern, and grammar school. The West German per capita educational expenditure is second only to the United States among the ten countries studied. The final grammar school certificate entitles the student to go to any institution of higher education. There are also full-time vocational schools for students who are 18 years or older. West Germany has the ninth highest secondary-school enrollment ratio in the world—at 90% for both male and females of secondary-school age. A relatively high proportion of older adolescents—57%—are in the labor force. Relatively few West German adolescents are married; only Japan has lower marriage rates among its adolescents.

West Germany is governed by a federal government whose members are elected. The parliament then elects the federal chancellor, who holds the power of head of government. There are three major political parties in West Germany.

The West Germany Sample was collected by Dr. Hans-Christoph Steinhausen, professor of child and adolescent psychiatry at the Free University of Berlin. His study provided data on 365 teenagers from four schools in the Charlottenburg District of central West Berlin, with ages ranging from 13 to 18. The students were from two high schools, a main school, and an intermediate school; one-third of the subjects were from lower-class families and the other two-thirds were from middle-class families. Letters were sent to the parents informing them of the research. The study was well accepted by both parents and teenagers. The German-language version of the OSIQ was administered to these subjects.

DATA ANALYSIS

Assuring Comparability of Translations of the OSIQ

A general problem in the use of questionnaires is that some respondents may not interpret a question in the way that the investigator intended. This problem is greatly exacerbated when the question is translated into other languages and interpreted in different cultural contexts. In considering the OSIQ from this point of view, we became acutely aware that many items contained colloquialisms (e.g., "carry grudges," "hit below the belt," "lose my head") that further complicated translation. Thus, each investigator was encouraged to create items that were as close as possible to the meaning of the original, rather than a literal translation of each word or phrase.

The original English-language version was used in only two samples—Australia and the United States. For the other eight countries, the OSIQ was translated into the appropriate language by the investigator or by a collaborator of the investigator. We used three methods to ensure the integrity of these translations.

The first method involved the use of back-translation. For each of the eight non-English-language versions of the OSIQ, we obtained a translation of that version into English. We then compared these back-translated items with the original OSIQ items. We sent the appropriate back-translated version to each investigator and discussed any apparent discrepancies. Correspondence continued until translation problems were resolved, or until scheduling forced the investigator into the field to collect data for his or her study (see Appendix 1 for the final back-translations of each item).

The second method utilized measures of the internal consistency of the 11 OSIQ scales for each country. Item-total correlations (corrected for item inclusion) were computed for each age-gender group for each country. Thus, for each item we obtained 38 estimates of the item-total correlation for each item (four age-gender groups from nine countries, two age-gender groups from Japan). An item was eliminated from a scale if it correlated negatively with the relevant scale score in more than four of the instances. Next, Cronbach alphas were computed for each scale for each country. If alphas were low across the four age-gender groups for any country, we identified items that also had low correlations with the scale total score for that country and eliminated the offending items from that scale for all countries.

Finally, we examined the endorsements for each item for each country. An item was eliminated from a scale if there was a unique pattern of endorsement for a country in conjunction with a questionable translation of that item as judged from the corresponding back-translation. For example, the back-translation of the Bengali version of the item "I feel relaxed under normal circumstances" was "Usually I feel very tired." The endorsement of this item in the Bengali sample was different from the endorsements of this item in all of the other countries. Consequently, this item was dropped for all countries.

As a result of these procedures, 26 items were eliminated from the 11 scales of the OSIQ. In addition, 6 items were eliminated because these items were not given in every country—some investigators used the second edition and others the third edition of the OSIQ (these two versions differ with respect to these 6 items). Since the Morals scale had very poor alphas, even after appropriate item elimination, that scale was entirely eliminated from the study. Deleting the Morals scale resulted in dropping 5 more items. Altogether, 31 items were eliminated. (Six items that were eliminated by the above procedure are included, separately, in some data analyses: Although these items could not be scored on any scale, they were endorsed consistently across age-gender groups across the ten countries, becoming part of what we call "universal" or universally endorsed items. They are listed under "individual" values.)

As a result of all these procedures the "international" version of the OSIQ comprises 99 items, 93 of which are combined into ten scales, as follows (number of items in parentheses):

Psychological Self-1:	Impulse Control Scale (7)
Psychological Self-2:	Emotional Tone Scale (9)
Psychological Self-3:	Body Image Scale (8)
Social Self-1:	Social Relationships Scale (9)
Social Self-2:	Morals (eliminated)
Social Self-3:	Vocational and Educational Goals Scale (7)
Sexual Self:	Sexual Attitudes Scale (9)
Familial Self:	Family Relationships Scale (18)
Coping Self-1:	Mastery of the External World Scale (5)
Coping Self-2:	Psychopathology Scale (10)
Coping Self-3:	Superior Adjustment Scale (11)

The alphas (internal consistencies) for these scales are shown in Appendix 2.

Analysis of the OSIQ

There were five foci of our analyses of teenagers' responses to the OSIQ. The first concerned the identification of responses that were characteristic of adolescents across countries—universal items. The second involved the determination of consistent age or gender differences across countries. Third, we investigated cross-national differences in self-image at both the scale and item levels. Fourth, we developed a measure of depression among teenagers and compared the extent of depression among adolescents in the various countries studied. The fifth analysis concerned the extent to which OSIQ scale score differences among countries were associated with economic and demographic characteristics of the countries.

Universal Items

The structured response format for each item of the OSIQ ranges from 1 ("describes me very well") to 6 ("does not describe me at all"). A response of 1, 2, or 3 represents an endorsement of the item. A response of 4, 5, or 6 represents a negation of that item. For each item, percent endorsements were calculated for each age-gender group for each country. This procedure yielded 38 endorsement percentages for each item (four age-gender groups for nine countries, older boys and older girls for Japan). An item was considered "universal" if at least 37 of the 38 endorsement percentages were 75% or above and no value was below 67%. An item also was considered "universal" if it was universally negated—that is, if at least 37 of the 38 endorsement percentages for that item were 25% or less and no value was above 33%. In this way we identified 16 items that were "universal" across the ten countries. The description and discussion of these items appears in Chapter 4.

Age and Gender Differences

In order to investigate consistent gender or age differences across countries, a three-way multivariate analysis of variance was performed. The independent variables in this analysis were age (younger—13 through 15, or older—16 through 19), gender, and country (nine countries, excluding Japan). The dependent variables were the ten OSIQ scale scores for each subject. The results of this analysis showed many statistically significant main effects of age, gender, and country, but no significant interaction effects.

We further explored the results of the univariate three-way analyses of variance of each of the ten OSIQ scales in this way: If there was a significant main effect for gender and/or age, we inspected the difference between the two means (boys versus girls, younger versus older) to determine if the algebraic sign of these differences was consistent across the nine countries. For those scales where there was a significant main effect and the differences were consistent across countries, we examined percent endorsement differences between boys and girls and/or between younger and older teenagers for the items in that scale. Interpretations were made if the age or gender differences were consistent across all nine countries. Results and discussion of these analyses appear in Chapter 4.

Cross-National Differences in Adolescent Self-Image

Differences at the Scale Score Level. Nine countries were used for these analyses (Japan was not included because data with respect to younger Japanese adolescents were not available). The three-way analyses of variance described above yielded a significant main effect for country for every OSIQ scale. To explore the meaning of these cross-national comparisons, whether a country's teenagers were high or low on each OSIQ scale was determined as follows: The ranking of each country's adolescents for each age-by-gender group on each OSIQ scale was calculated. A country's teenagers were considered high or low on a scale if they were consistently in the top third or bottom third of the countries studied across all four age-by-sex cells—that is, younger males, younger females, older males, and older females. To illustrate, for each age-gender group, the nine countries were rank-ordered for positiveness of self-image with respect to Impulse Control. Across the four age-gender groups, Hungarian adolescents were consistently in the top third and Italian adolescents were consistently in the lowest third with respect to this scale. Since for any age-gender group in a country there is a 1-in-3 probability (ranking first, second, or third among the nine countries) by chance alone of being among the top third of the countries studied on any scale, there is only a 1-in-81 probability by chance alone of that country's being among the top third across all four age-by-gender groups—similarly for the bottom third.

Differences at the Item Level. An item was selected as consistently high or low if (a) it occurred on a scale showing at least one consistent intercountry difference (a country consistently in the top third or bottom third of the nine countries studied on the scale for all four age-gender groups), and (b) a country in the top (or bottom) third for all four groups for the *scale* was also in the top (or bottom) third for all four groups with respect to that *item.* Thus, Bangladesh was in the bottom third among the countries studied in all four age-gender groups with respect to Impulse Control. With respect to item 17, which is part of this scale, Bangladesh was in the bottom third in all four cells. Thus, item 17 was selected for exposition. Other items for this and other scales were considered similarly. Occasionally we will discuss items that do not have consistent cross-national differences because they are of special interest.

Depression among Adolescents

The depression scale (see Chapter 4) was constructed as follows: As a first step, we searched the OSIQ for items that would reflect depression—that is, chronic sadness, loneliness, and emptiness. Five items were selected as indicators of depression (items 45, 61, 66, 103, and 130). A depression score was calculated by adding the responses to the five items for each subject. In order to check the psychometric integrity of this scale, measures of internal consistency—item-total correlations and alphas—were computed for each age-gender group for each country. Inspection revealed good internal consistency for this scale (see Appendix 4 for a display of the alphas).

In addition, percent endorsements were ascertained for each age-gender-country group. Since the depression scale comprises five items, scores could range from 5 ("describes me very well" for each of the five items after appropriate reversing) to 30 ("does not describe me at all" for each of the five items after appropriate reversing). A score of 15 or lower on this scale represents an average response on the affirmative side (3 or less for each of the five items); as a result, a score of 15 or lower was considered an "endorsement" of depression.

Economic and Demographic Correlates of Self-Image

Although our emphasis is on characteristics of self-image that are consistent across countries, we were also interested in correlates of difference among countries. For this purpose we selected 18 economic and demographic characteristics for exploration. These were as follows:

- Gross national product (GNP)
- Per capita income
- Population density
- Percent living in urban areas
- Index of net social progress (based on 55 variables)
- Physical quality of life index (life expectancy, infant mortality, literacy)
- Number of TV sets per 1,000 individuals
- Percent of 14- to 18-year-olds in total population
- Percent of GNP spent on education
- Per capita expenditure for education
- Percent of students enrolled in secondary schools
- Postsecondary-school enrollment per 1,000 students
- Percent of 15- to 19-year-old females in the labor force
- Percent of 15- to 19-year-old males in the labor force
- Marriage rate among 15- to 19-year-old males per 1,000
- Marriage rate among 15- to 19-year-old females per 1,000
- Birth rate among 15- to 19-year-old mothers per 1,000
- Divorce rate among 15- to 19-year-olds

For each OSIQ scale, for each of the four age-gender groups, the nine countries (excluding Japan) were rank-ordered on the basis of mean scale scores. Similarly, the countries were rank-ordered with respect to each of the economic and demographic characteristics. Rank-order correlations $(N = 9)$ were calculated between each OSIQ scale and each demographic characteristic. If the correlation between a scale score and an economic and demographic characteristic was statistically significant for at least three age-gender groups, the association was interpreted. The results and discussion of these analyses appear in Chapter 4.

Let us turn now to the major part of this book—the results of our empirical investigations. The 5,938 adolescents from the ten countries are the ones who supplied us with their feelings and thoughts, and allowed us to enter their inner psychological world. Hence, what we are reporting in the next chapter is not our interpretation of what they said. Rather, it is what they said.

Results of Data Analysis
A Study of 5938 Adolescents in Ten Countries

Universal Aspects of the Adolescent Experience • *Gender Differences in Adolescent Self-Image* • *Age Differences in Adolescent Self-Image* • *Cross-National Scale and Item Differences* • *Depression or Quiet Disturbance among Adolescents* • *Demography, the Economy, and Adolescent Self-Image*

UNIVERSAL ASPECTS OF THE ADOLESCENT EXPERIENCE

Across the ten countries studied, teenagers showed broad agreement. This agreement was concentrated in family relationships, vocational and educational goals, superior adjustment (or coping), social relationships, and, to a limited extent, individual values (see Table 1).

Familial Self

Items measuring family relationships showed the most agreement across countries. The overwhelming majority of teenagers in all ten countries disclaimed negative attitudes toward their families. To illustrate, over 91% of teenagers in each country denied carrying a grudge against their parents. The vast majority denied feeling that either their mother (91%) or their father (87%) is no good. Teenagers do not believe that their parents are ashamed of them (93%) or that their parents will be disappointed in them in the future (89%). About 82% of the teenagers studied in the various countries stated that their parents get along well with each other.

The lack of negativity of these attitudes contrasts with popular and professional conceptions of adolescents as alienated from their parents—conceptions that emphasize turmoil and the "generation gap."

TABLE 1. Universal Items: Positive Endorsements[a]

Items	Average percentage endorsement[b]
Positive endorsements	
Social relationships	
88. Being together with other people gives me a good feeling.	88
Vocational and educational goals	
58. At times I think about what kind of work I will do in the future.	90
70. A job well done gives me pleasure.	96
79. I feel that there is plenty I can learn from others.	89
Family relationships	
51. Most of the time my parents get along well with each other.	82
Superior adjustment	
84. If I know that I will have to face a new situation, I will try in advance to find out as much as is possible about it.	85
89. Whenever I fail in something, I try to find out what I can do in order to avoid another failure.	87
Individual values	
83. I like to help a friend whenever I can.	92
Negative endorsements	
Vocational and educational goals	
63. I would rather be supported for the rest of my life than work	10
Family relationships	
95. My parents are ashamed of me.	7
106. I have been carrying a grudge against my parents for years.	9
118. Very often I feel that my mother is no good.	9
15. My parents will be disappointed in me in the future.	11
21. Very often I feel that my father is no good.	13
Superior adjustment	
107. I am certain that I will not be able to assume responsibilities for myself in the future.	12
Individual values	
48. Telling the truth means nothing to me.	15

[a] In order to qualify as "universal," an item must have an average endorsement of 75% or more within each country and none of the four groups (e.g., younger males) can have less than 67% endorsement.
[b] The percentage endorsements were averaged across all four cells (gender and age) across all countries.

Instead, it seems that adolescents are in the mainstream of their parents' values. They accept and esteem their parents and feel that these attitudes are reciprocated.

Social Self

Another area generating universal agreement among teenagers concerned vocational and educational goals. Adolescents affirmed the value of work and their interest in it. This affirmation is reflected in the fact that 90% reported that they think about the kind of work they will do in the future. Ninety-six percent stated that a job well done gives them pleasure. The vast majority of adolescents indicated that they have much to learn from other people (89%). In the same vein, 90% of the adolescents we studied denied that they would rather be supported for the rest of their lives than work.

These results contrast with a view of teenagers as self-centered and directionless. Adolescents want to work and derive pleasure from working. Moreover, they are willing to look toward other people for guidance.

Other items indicate that adolescents are interpersonally and peer-oriented. In addition, they affirm high moral values. Eighty-eight percent of teenagers stated that being together with other people gives them a good feeling. Ninety-two percent stated that they like to help a friend whenever then can. Indicating the moral standards of teenagers, only 15% reported that telling the truth means nothing to them. Seeing adolescents as simply self-centered and disrespectful is contraindicated by these results.

Coping Self

Adolescents also report good coping skills. They relate that when they fail at something, they try to find out what they can do about it in order to avoid another failure (87%). If they have to face a new situation, they will try to find out as much as possible about it in advance (85%). Only 12% of the teenagers felt that they will not be able to assume responsibility for themselves in the future. Thus, teenagers not only affirm work-related values, they relate having the skills to accomplish what they set out to do. Once again, the image teenagers have of themselves contrasts with a view of them as floundering, impulse-ridden, and oriented only to immediate gratification.

In sum, it is the positive aspects of their experience upon which teenagers in countries widely distributed throughout the world agree. A discussion of these findings follows.

    As we found in earlier studies, which were centered on American
adolescents, teenagers are family-oriented. All teenagers must, to one
degree or another, change their relationship with their family of origin.
In Western cultures, this change usually entails leaving one's family of
origin both physically and psychologically, becoming increasingly invested in peer relationships, and ultimately becoming part of a new,
conjugal family. But teenagers' changing their relationship with their
family of origin is different from rebelling against or becoming antag-
onistic toward that family. Theorists of adolescent functioning have
described rebellion and antagonism as a necessary step toward adolescents' separating from their parents and moving toward becoming parents in their own right. Our data suggest that, in countries throughout
the world, teenagers are able to become more independent from their
family of origin without bitterness or disavowal. They can express their
love and admiration for their parents while feeling comfortable with
forming relationships outside their immediate family. They feel confident that their parents approve of their growth and will be proud of
them in the future. From the teenager's point of view, the "generation
gap" is a myth conceived and nurtured in the minds of theoreticians.

    Also central to adolescent development is the formation of new
and expanded peer relationships. Friends facilitate teenagers' separating from their family of origin and help teenagers to discover their own
identity or place in the social network. Along with expressing positive
attitudes toward their family of origin, our data show that adolescents
affirm good feelings toward peers. Apparently, teenagers feel no conflict between good feelings toward their parents and good feelings toward their friends. They affirm the worth of both sets of people and are
not overwhelmed by their having to reach out to form new relationships. They feel good about these new relationships without having to
disavow the old.

    Another major task of adolescence concerns consolidating a work-
related identity. The industrial revolution created a need for extended
periods of training to qualify persons to perform technologically de-
manding roles. This process shapes the experience of middle-class
teenagers throughout the world. The teenagers we studied face acquir-
ing adult roles with confidence. They affirmed the value of and look
forward to work. The type of work they will perform in the future is of
great interest to adolescents: There is no indication in these data that
future work is a source of great concern and worry. The adolescents we
studied affirmed good coping skills. They expressed an understanding
that it is not enough to simply be oriented toward the future. Instead,
they agreed, one must benefit from what others have learned in the

past, learn from one's own mistakes, and prepare to the best of one's ability for future tasks.

It is of interest to note which self-image areas did not generate universal agreement. There was no universal agreement with respect to the psychological self—that is, impulse control, emotional tone, and body image—or the sexual self. The psychological self and the sexual self, as will be shown later, were much more a function of gender differences and socioeconomic variables than they were the subject of universal affirmation or denial. Apparently, what teenagers agree upon encompasses values, goals, and relationships. Mood, self-control, and body image vary much more widely as a function of circumstance. Sexual attitudes also are highly variable across groups and nations.

GENDER DIFFERENCES IN ADOLESCENT SELF-IMAGE

Gender-difference findings are striking in that perhaps for the first time extensive data are available showing contrasts between boys' and girls' self-image that are cross-national in scope (see Tables 2 and 3). These results do not reflect only local cultural phenomena.

Psychological Self Differences

Boys reported better control of their feelings, less emotional vulnerability, and a greater degree of happiness than did girls. They related more interest in and confidence about sexuality. They consistently expressed more pride in and positive feelings about their bodies.

In all ten countries, boys were more likely than were girls to portray themselves as being in control of the vicissitudes of their emotions. Seventy-one percent of the boys expressed ability to control emotional behavior such as crying and laughing, while only 53% of the girls did so. Eighty percent of the boys reported being able to keep an even temper most of the time, while 74% of the girls did so.

Boys, at a subjective level, seem to be better off than are girls. Across countries, adolescent males expressed a more positive sense of subjective well-being than did adolescent females. Thirty-four percent of the girls frequently feel sad; 25% of the boys frequently feel sad. Similarly, boys appeared to be more self-confident than did girls. For two-thirds of the boys, "our society is a competitive one, and I am not afraid of it." Fifty-seven percent of the girls endorsed this item.

The area of body image contains particularly striking contrasts between boys' and girls' self-image. A much higher percent of the boys

TABLE 2. Items Endorsed More Often by Boys Than by Girls
across the Ten Countries[a]

Items	Average percentage endorsement[b]	
	Male	Female
Impulse control		
69. I keep an even temper most of the time.	80	74
Emotional tone		
68. I enjoy life.	83	80
Body image		
42. The picture I have of myself in the future satisfies me.	70	66
57. I am proud of my body.	67	52
Vocational and educational goals		
46. I would rather sit around and loaf than work.	29	22
63. I would rather be supported for the rest of my life than work.	14	7
115. School and studying mean very little to me.	21	15
Sexual attitudes		
28. Dirty jokes are fun at times.	67	52
117. Sexual experiences give me pleasure.	72	44
122. I often think about sex.	63	40
Family relationships		
51. Most of the time my parents get along well with each other.	84	80
Superior adjustment		
49. Our society is a competitive one and I am not afraid of it.	68	57
Individual values		
67. I do not care how my actions affect others as long as I gain something.	22	14

[a] Must be minimum of 16 of 19 comparisons with the sex difference in the same direction. Sixteen represents odds of ($p < .001$) based on a mean of 9.5 and an SD of $\sqrt{n\,p(1-p)} = \sqrt{19(1/2)(1/2)} = 2.18$; $16 = 9.5 + (3)(2.18) = \bar{X} + 3\ SD$.
[b] Average of the percent endorsements (rounded off to the nearest whole) for each gender for the ten countries.

(67%) than of the girls (52%) expressed being proud of their bodies. Across ten countries, girls much more often reported feeling ugly and unattractive than did boys. Thirty-eight percent of the girls and 27% of the boys reported feeling this way. It should be noted that these differences are not confined to early age groups. If they were, it could be argued that results are a function of girls' going through puberty at an earlier age on the average than do boys. Girls' responses could then be interpreted as a function of their responding in a negative way to a rapidly growing and changing body. But male–female differences in body image hold during later adolescence as well—during a time when it is the boys who are experiencing more rapid body changes. As a result, it is more likely that sociological, historical, and psychological factors, not biological factors, account for differences in male–female disparities in body image.

TABLE 3. *Items Endorsed More Often by Girls Than by Boys across the Ten Countries*[a]

Items	Average percentage endorsement[b]	
	Female	Male
Impulse control		
17. At times I have fits of crying and/or laughing that I seem unable to control.	47	29
81. I fear something constantly.	35	29
Emotional tone		
38. My feelings are easily hurt.	62	44
130. I frequently feel sad.	34	25
Body image		
82. Very often I think that I am not at all the person I would like to be.	48	40
90. I frequently feel ugly and unattractive.	38	27
Sexual attitudes		
80. I do not attend sexy shows.	67	47
91. Sexually I am way behind.	22	16
Psychopathology		
22. I am confused most of the time.	35	27
36. Sometimes I feel so ashamed of myself that I just want to hide in a corner and cry.	31	21
61. I often feel that I would rather die than go on living.	24	18
Superior adjustment		
39. When a tragedy occurs to one of my friends I feel sad too.	94	83
Individual values		
83. I like to help a friend whenever I can.	94	90

[a] Must be minimum of 16 of 19 comparisons with the sex difference in the same direction. Sixteen represents odds of $(p < .001)$ based on a mean of 9.5 and an SD of $\sqrt{n\,p(1-p)} = \sqrt{19(1/2)(1/2)} = 2.18$; $16 = 9.5 + (3)(2.18) = \bar{X}\ 3\ SD$.
[b] Average of the percent endorsements (rounded off to the nearest whole) for each gender for the ten countries.

Sexual Self Differences

Across the ten nations studied, boys expressed much more interest in and positive feelings about sexuality. A larger proportion of the boys (63%) than of the girls (40%) reported that they frequently think about sex. Two-thirds of the girls denied attending sexy shows; only 47% of the boys did so. Boys were more likely to affirm that dirty jokes are fun at times (67% vs. 52%). Seventy-two percent of the boys and only 44% of the girls reported that sexual experiences give them pleasure. Girls' less positive feelings about sexuality probably stems from traditional attitudes toward female sexuality. At least in the Western tradition, attitudes toward sexuality seem to have waxed more or less conservative throughout various historical periods. But even in this tradition it is not attitudes toward male sexuality that have tended to change. Instead, attitudes toward female sexuality have become more or less permissive, with greater permissiveness toward female sexuality in eras such as the early industrial age in England and the Roaring Twenties, and less permissiveness in the Victorian age and the post-1960s–1970s era in modern America. In all the societies studied, girls' sexuality is the subject of greater control and concern than is boys' sexuality.

Social Self Differences

In contrast to boys, girls report a higher degree of social awareness and commitment to others. Their stance is more sociable and empathic. To cite one example, 94% of the girls, as opposed to 83% of the boys, related feeling sad when a tragedy occurs to one of their friends. Across all ten countries, girls were more likely to report feeling that they like to help a friend whenever they can. In contrast, a larger proportion of the boys (22%) than of the girls (14%) endorsed the item "I do not care how my actions affect others as long as I gain something." Perhaps related to girls' more sociable and empathic stance is the fact that across all the samples girls were more likely than were boys to report that their parents do not get along well with each other. There seems to be no clear reason why the parents of girls would not get along as well as the parents of boys except perhaps that girls may simply be more sensitive than boys to intrafamilial conflict, and more involved with their families. Girls are thus in a better position to be aware of or sensitive to any conflict that might be present (e.g., Harris and Howard, 1985).

Girls, in addition, expressed more commitment to the work ethic, including investment in school and studying. Twenty-one percent of the girls (vs. 15% of the boys) denied feeling that school and studying mean very little to them. Across all ten samples, girls were less likely to report feeling they would rather sit around and loaf than work. Twice as many boys as girls (14% vs. 7%) endorsed wanting to be supported for the rest of their lives rather than work. It is of interest that in this area boys' self-image does not conform to the stereotype of confident and self-sufficient masculinity. It is the girls who express commitment to the desirability of effort and achievement. The boys' position is more self-centered and self-indulgent.

When trying to appreciate these findings, a central issue is the accuracy of the boys' and girls' self-report. By way of illustration, consider boys' reporting less frequent feelings of sadness than did the girls. The simplest explanation is that the boys are in fact less sad than are the girls. Another explanation is that boys are less aware of feelings of sadness than are girls. In other words, they may not be as introspective as the girls and, in general, may be more uncomfortable with feelings. This issue falls under the rubric of social desirability, a central issue in self-report measurement. For many years psychologists have struggled with whether an individual's response to an item on a questionnaire reflects that individual's true feelings or whether the response reflects the individual's perception of what the socially desirable ("right") response is. The act of giving responses that are essentially just socially desirable need not be a deliberate one. Respondents could believe that they are the way they should be and give responses that reflect that belief rather than an underlying psychological reality. Following these models, boys might less frequently attest to feelings of sadness because they might believe that reporting sadness would cast them in a less masculine—that is, less socially desirable—light. Or they might believe that however negative their feelings are, those feelings could not be termed "sadness" because under ordinary circumstances men should not feel sad. Another possibility is that all these factors are simultaneously operative: Boys are less sad, they resist admitting they are sad to others, and they tend not to acknowledge sad feelings they may have, even to themselves.

Our methodology militated against the influence of social desirability because the OSIQ was administered under anonymous conditions. It seems less likely that subjects would deliberately express socially desirable as opposed to actual feelings when they know that they will never individually be associated with the responses that they have given. In some ways, however, the issue regarding the socially desirable, as opposed to the authentic, nature of responses is both moot and unsolvable. It is unsolvable because, unless subjects are manifesting clinically observable symptomatology, such as weeping or insomnia, these subjects' feelings are not directly or at least reliably observable, with the result that the subjects' self-reports present the only way an observer can learn about their affectual state. If one were to set aside self-report as a source of knowledge about subjects' actual feelings because that self-report might be a function of social desirability, then the subjects' actual feelings could never be known. It is moot because from a behavioral point of view it is as important to know the characteristics presented by the subjects out of a sense of social desirability as it is to know the true underlying feelings and attitudes of those subjects. Both the subjects' ideas of what is socially desirable and their true underlying feelings and attitudes will be determinative of their behavior. Thus, knowing either one will be an important source of data. Whether boys actually feel less sad or are less prone to admit to feeling sad may not be as important as the fact that they indicate they are not sad and the behavioral consequences that flow from that indication.

In this spirit, let us consider these alternative ways of construing our results. In one scenario, boys feel impelled to present themselves as controlled, confident, and self-centered human beings; they describe themselves as both opportunistic and happy; they relate being sexually liberal and proud of their bodies. Girls feel impelled to present themselves as emotionally expressive and vulnerable; they more often relate self-doubt, particularly in the area of body image; they describe themselves as sociable and empathic and committed to traditional values.

Another possibility is that boys and girls accurately portray their underlying feelings. In this scenario, boys in fact feel more in control, happier, and more self-confident than do girls. Girls in reality are more sociable and committed to traditional values. Compared to boys, girls more frequently feel ugly and unattractive and are not as proud of their bodies. In either case, explanations of these differences are almost certainly primarily historical and social. Such explanations are necessarily speculative, but they most likely center around the different historical and social roles played by males and females in the societies we studied: What is most startling about our findings is the consistency in differences in boys' and girls' self-image across the ten nations studied. If historical and social explanations are relevant, then these explanations cannot invoke circumstances that are unique to only one or a few of the nations we studied. The explanations must concern factors that exist or existed in all ten of these disparate nations. What the data seem to show most clearly is that among 1980s samples of young persons, gender differences in self-image seem most closely related to traditional sex roles. If boys do in fact feel more in control, happier, and more self-confident than do girls, the reason may be linked to the role that societies traditionally hold out for them, roles that are associated with greater power and access to resources than those available to women. An analogous explanation would hold for the girls' greater commitment to traditional values and their greater sociability. As noted earlier, women are traditionally more invested in interpersonal relationships and affective bonding, particularly in the immediate family unit, than are men. The relatively poor body image of girls may relate to their low self-confidence on the one hand, and the importance of being attractive in order to achieve traditional female goals of marriage and children on the other. As we explained in an earlier book (Offer, Ostrov, and Howard, 1981a), attractiveness is often felt to be a biological given rather than an achieved status. Girls often feel that attractiveness is an important component of their ability to attract and keep a mate, and also to achieve status with their peers. The need to attract and keep a mate heightens the importance of being physically attractive. Not being able to achieve attractiveness through effort heightens the feeling of vulnerability with respect to this area of life. Low self-confidence— perhaps associated with the relatively low status of females in societies throughout the world—ensures that feeling vulnerable with respect to attractiveness results in concern and even belief that one is ugly and unattractive.

AGE DIFFERENCES IN ADOLESCENT SELF-IMAGE

In general, we found that older adolescents are more self-confident than are younger adolescents. They express being more open to the feelings and opinions of others. These results are consistent with expectations and both expound upon the nature of development during the adolescent period and help confirm the validity of using self-report as a way of investigating the psychological functioning of teenagers (see Tables 4 and 5).

Across all ten countries older adolescents were more likely than were younger adolescents to report feeling "there is plenty that I can learn from others." Sixty-six percent of the older adolescents, but only 60% of the younger adolescents, expressed being able to take criticism without resentment.

From a psychological point of view, being able to learn from others and take criticism without resentment is evidence of self-confidence and what could be called "healthy narcissism." Being able to take criticism without feeling diminished in a painful or even devastating way shows an accumulation of positive self-esteem. Criticism occurs in the context of positive self-feelings with the result that it is experienced as enhancing rather than destructive. Other persons are not experienced simply as rivals to be bested or defeated at all costs. Individuals

TABLE 4. *Items Endorsed More Often by Younger Adolescents Than by Older Adolescents across the Nine Countries*[a]

	Average percentage endorsement[b]	
Items	Younger	Older
Body image		
94. When others look at me they must think that I am poorly developed.	17	13
Sexual attitudes		
97. Thinking or talking about sex scares me.	21	13
Family relationships		
9. My parents are almost always on the side of someone else, for example, my brother or sister.	29	22
51. Most of the time my parents get along well with each other.	85	79
Psychopathology		
2. When I am with people I am afraid that someone will make fun of me.	27	22

[a] Must be minimum of 15 of 18 comparisons with the age difference in the same direction. Fifteen represents odds of ($p < .005$) based on a mean of 9 and an SD of $\sqrt{n\,p(1-p)} = \sqrt{18(1/2)(1/2)} = 2.12$; $\bar{X} + 3\,SD = 15.36$.

[b] Average of the percent endorsements (rounded off to the nearest whole) for each age group for the nine countries (excluding Japan).

who are confident and have positive self-esteem can acknowledge the worth of others without feeling a devastating loss in their own self-esteem. Our data suggest that the course of development during adolescence is a positive one. As they become older, adolescents are more able to learn from others and more able to accept criticism than are younger adolescents, and older adolescents reflect increasing accumulation of positive self-esteem and confidence.

Another finding is that across countries a higher percentage of younger adolescents as compared to older adolescents express that when they are with people they feel afraid someone will make fun of them. Twenty-seven percent of younger teenagers and 22% of older teenagers endorsed this item across the countries studied. Younger adolescents (17%) are more likely than are older adolescents (13%) to feel that "when others look at me, they must think that I am poorly developed." Self-consciousness is one of the hallmarks of young adolescence. The experience of young adolescents often is that when other people observe them, those others receive a negative impression of

TABLE 5. *Items Endorsed More Often by Older Adolescents Than by Younger Adolescents across the Ten Countries*[a]

	Average percentage endorsement[b]	
Items	Younger	Older
Impulse control		
34. I can take criticism without resentment.	60	66
Vocational and educational goals		
79. I feel that there is plenty I can learn from others.	86	90
Sexual attitudes		
117. Sexual experiences give me pleasure.	51	66

[a] Must be minimum of 15 of 18 comparisons with the age difference in the same direction. Fifteen represents odds of ($p < .005$) based on a mean of 9 and an SD of $\sqrt{n\,p(1-p)} = \sqrt{18(1/2)(1/2)} = 2.12$; $\bar{X} + 3\,SD = 15.36$.
[b] Average of the percent endorsements (rounded off to the nearest whole) for each age group for the ten countries.

them. As a result, young adolescents often try to avoid this experience. An explanation can be given in cognitive terms. The beginning of adolescence is marked by increased exposure to and concern with peers. These peers often present points of view that are at variance with those experienced by adolescents in their own families. At the same time, young adolescents become more capable of thinking of themselves from the point of view of other people (Piaget, 1967). At the beginning of adolescence, therefore, there is both an increase in awareness that one is the object of others' opinions and an increase in knowledge that others' opinions may be very different from one's own. As a result there is a surge of doubt and concern as to whether one is living up to the expectations of others. This self-awareness and self-doubt occurs in the context of relatively little experience with feedback from others, particularly nonfamily members, as to one's relative self-worth. As a result, any negative feedback is weighty in proportion to the total amount of feedback that that adolescent has received. If someone makes fun of a young adolescent, that mockery occurs against a background of relatively few positive affirmations of self. As a result, such mockery can be relatively destructive and is something to fear and avoid. In contrast, older persons who have had a great deal of positive feedback about themselves will be less vulnerable to any single instance of negative criticism. Thus, it can be predicted—if the general course of adolescence is to accumulate positive feedback about oneself—that older adolescents will feel less afraid of criticism or mockery from others. Our data suggest that this is exactly what does occur during adolescence.

Older adolescents seem to have a more balanced view of their families than do younger adolescents. Thus, a larger proportion of younger than older adolescents (29% vs. 22%) related that their parents are partial to some other individual, such as a brother or a sister.

It is likely that young adolescents' view of their parents' partiality is a function not of their parents in fact being more partial but of young adolescents' relatively low self-confidence. A person with relatively low self-confidence is likely to assimilate experiences to a negative view of himself in the world and interpret any slight as confirming that view. To a young adolescent, a parent's giving something to a brother or sister might be experienced as showing that they have more positive feelings toward that brother or sister. A more self-confident older adolescent might experience that same act of giving to a brother or a sister as a statement about the parents' feelings toward their children, not as an act somehow negatively directed toward him or her.

Older adolescents were more likely to relate being comfortable with sexual feelings and experiences than were younger adolescents. Sixty-six percent of older adolescents and 51% of younger adolescents reported that sexual experiences give them pleasure. A larger proportion of younger than of older adolescents (21% vs. 13%) reported that "thinking or talking about sex scares me."

The simplest explanation of these findings is that sex, for most young adolescents, is unexplored territory that, like any unknown, leads to feelings of apprehension. It can be expected that for many young adolescents sex is not so much intriguing as it is yet another source of self-doubt. What probably is scary for many young adolescents about sex is that this is one more area that they have to try to do well at—or at least not fail at—or is one more area of unknown risks. With experience comes confidence, and, across the nations studied, older adolescents, who almost certainly are more sexually experienced than are younger adolescents in every nation, are more likely to report more ability to derive pleasure from and less apprehension about sex.

It is of interest that younger adolescents were more likely than were older adolescents to express feeling that their parents get along well with each other. Younger teenagers' feeling that their parents get along well may be more reflective of their lack of sensitivity to and involvement with their family. These teenagers still have the child's conception of an idealized parental pair that prevents them from seeing their parents as they really are. In addition, they may be too involved with their peer culture to notice what is going on in the home.

In general, the results reported in this section were consistent with our expectations. Almost all developmental psychologists would agree that adolescence encompasses a process of increasing maturity, knowledgeability, and self-confidence. Not experiencing this kind of growth would represent a failure of this period of development. Our data simply captured the universality of this experience. At the same time, they show the meaningfulness of self-report. Older adolescents experience and are able to report their greater confidence and maturity. They flesh out what that means to them: being able to listen to and learn from others, being able to profit from criticism, being confident enough to be with others without fear of being demeaned. Younger adolescents are able to describe their relative insecurity or lack of maturity: the fear of mockery, the sensitivity to criticism or emotional deprivation, and the apprehension regarding future experiences such as sexuality.

CROSS-NATIONAL SCALE AND ITEM DIFFERENCES

In this section we highlight some of the differences we found among the teenagers from the ten different countries. We need to keep in mind that the similarities between our subjects considerably outweighed their differences. Yet differences across countries are of interest and have ramifications concerning the cross-national study and developmental psychology of adolescents.

Psychological Self

Impulse Control

Two countries, Bangladesh and Italy, were consistently low on this scale (Table 6). No country was consistently high on impulse control. Item analyses showed that 65% of Bengali youths reported that at times they feel like laughing or crying so hard that they cannot stop. This rate is double that of most of the other countries. Many (42%) Bengali youths reported constantly feeling afraid. Only Taiwanese youths endorsed this item at a higher rate. The apparent poor impulse control of Italian youths may be, to a degree, a function of their failure to endorse one item, "I keep an even temper most of the time" (item 69), at a relatively high rate. That item, however, may have been poorly translated. The Italian item when back-translated into English was "I am almost always in a bad humor." Italian youths' not affirming this item is understandable and would not necessarily imply lack of impulse

TABLE 6. *Psychological Self: Items within Each Self Showing Consistent Intercountry Differences across Age and Gender*[a]

No.	Item	Percent endorsement								
		Australia	Bangladesh	Hungary	Israel	Italy	Taiwan	Turkey	United States	West Germany
12.	I feel tense most of the time.	26	63	23	24	32	49	50	26	30
17.	At times I have fits of crying and/or laughing that I seem unable to control.	44	65	33	31	38	31	39	38	28
23.	I feel inferior to most people I know.	27	33	10	14	19	25	20	17	8
27.	In the past year I have been very worried about my health.	29	56	15	19	29	37	23	31	18
38.	My feelings are easily hurt.	52	69	27	63	55	44	65	59	41
42.	The picture I have of myself in the future satisfies me.	69	88	59	77	76	68	53	88	61
57.	I am proud of my body.	56	59	41	73	68	62	62	76	68
66.	I feel so very lonely.	22	43	14	17	20	33	31	19	11
68.	I enjoy life.	83	69	82	88	91	71	86	92	85
69.	I keep an even temper most of the time.	72	72	78	82	64	90	77	84	82
72.	I seem to be forced to imitate the people I like.	29	64	37	28	24	59	24	27	12
81.	I fear something constantly.	37	42	18	27	42	58	29	23	11
82.	Very often I think that I am not at all the person I would like to be.	53	54	44	28	38	50	41	39	28
90.	I frequently feel ugly and unattractive.	36	37	30	27	34	28	29	27	18
94.	When others look at me they must think that I am poorly developed.	16	30	11	15	8	20	21	12	4
99.	I feel strong and healthy.	74	48	80	86	78	55	87	89	80
123.	Usually I control myself.	85	81	83	88	78	67	87	92	69
130.	I frequently feel sad.	27	37	24	27	25	25	33	23	17

[a] Items presented (1) were on a scale on which at least one country was consistently high (or low) in all four age-by-gender cells and (2) were consistently high (or low) for that country for that scale. Consistently high (or low) was defined in terms of being in the upper (or lower) third of nine countries in all four age-by-gender cells. Percentages shown are the average percent endorsement for that item for the country across four age-by-gender cells.

control. However, Italian youths did report relatively poor impulse control with respect to one adequately translated item, "Usually I control myself" (77%, the third lowest endorsement rate).

Emotional Tone

Hungarian youths consistently ranked in the top third on this scale. Bengali youths consistently ranked poorest. Item analyses showed that Bengali youths ranked poorest because a relatively large proportion (63%) attested to feeling a "mental pressure" most of the time. They endorsed feeling "inferior to many people I know" at a higher rate than did youths from any other country. Bengali youths showed relatively high endorsement of being "easily hurt" (69%), feeling "very lonely" (43%), and "frequently [being] weighed down with sadness" (37%). Bengali adolescents also were less likely to attest to enjoying life than were other youths (69%, the lowest endorsement rate across countries for this item).

The relatively good emotional functioning attested to by Hungarian adolescents was due in good measure to a single item. In the original, the item read, "My feelings are easily hurt." The back-translation from the Hungarian was "I am easily offended." Hungarian teenagers' relatively low-level endorsement of that item (27% vs. 41% for the next lowest country) might represent a somewhat different meaning of the item when translated. With respect to other items on this scale, the pattern showed by the Hungarian youths tended to be age-specific rather than consistent across groups. Among younger Hungarian adolescents there were very positive attestations, while older adolescents showed less positive endorsement rates. (The relatively poorer functioning of older as opposed to younger Hungarian adolescents has been explicated by Kertész, Offer, Ostrov, and Howard, 1986.) To illustrate, younger Hungarian adolescents endorsed feeling tense at a much lower rate than did younger adolescents from any other country. Older Hungarian adolescents were average in their endorsement rate for this item. Younger Hungarian boys endorsed the item "most of the time I am happy" at a high rate, though not at as high a rate as Taiwanese or Israeli younger male adolescents; younger Hungarian girls endorsed this item at the highest rate among all the countries studied. But older Hungarian adolescents showed one of the lowest endorsement rates with respect to this item. With respect to the item "I feel sad often," younger Hungarian adolescents presented among the lowest levels of endorsement of any of the countries studied. In contrast, older Hungarian adolescents showed average-level endorsement rates (see Appendix 1).

Body Image

United States and German teenagers consistently reported the best body image. Bengali and Taiwanese youths consistently reported the poorest. American youths consistently reported higher levels of endorsement for the item "I am proud of my body"; 76% of American youths endorsed this item. The vast majority of German youths (82%) denied feeling "ugly and unattractive." Ninety-six percent of German youths denied that "when other people look at me they must feel that I am not very developed." American youths were consistently among the highest of those studied in their endorsement of "I feel strong and healthy"; 89% of American youths endorsed this item.

In contrast, many (37% and 56%, respectively) Taiwanese and Bengali adolescents related feeling "very worried about my health" in the past few years. Less than half the Bengali teenagers endorsed feeling "strong and healthy." Fifty-five percent of the Taiwanese teenagers did so. Far more Bengali youths (30%) reported that "when others see me, they must think that my physical form is not good" than did youths from other countries.

To summarize, in the area of the psychological self, Bengali adolescents consistently reported the lowest levels of functioning. Bengali teenagers are more lonely, sad, and vulnerable. They feel more afraid. Compared to teenagers from other countries, Bengali youths are less likely to endorse feeling strong and healthy. Relative lack of emotional control also was attested to by Bengali adolescents at relatively high rates. Taiwanese adolescents were almost as likely to be negative in their appraisal of their physical well-being and attractiveness as were the Bengali adolescents. In contrast, Hungarian adolescents, particularly younger Hungarian adolescents, were very positive in the psychological self endorsements. The relatively good emotional functioning of Hungarian adolescents, however, seems to diminish with age in comparison to the other groups of adolescents. United States and German teenagers tend to describe their feelings about their bodies in relatively positive terms.

One explanation for these results centers on economic conditions and opportunities experienced by teenagers in the different countries. Bengali teenagers live in an extremely poor country and do not have the economic advantages possessed by teenagers in industrialized countries such as the United States and Hungary. It could be argued that well-being is relative, and that these Bengali teenagers, compared to other adolescents in their country, may be extremely well off. Nevertheless, our results suggest that Bengali middle-class teenagers are not psychologically advantaged. The psychologically most advantaged teenagers in our study were those from Germany, Hungary, and the United States. Consistent with what may be a cultural emphasis on sports and physical development, industrialization probably has an effect in this area as well—with American and German teenagers more likely to feel healthy and proud of their bodies because they have available to them resources to take good care of themselves.

Social Self

Social Relationships

Two countries showed consistent rankings with respect to social relationships (Table 7). Hungarian adolescents consistently showed the highest while Bengali adolescents consistently showed the lowest rates of endorsement of good social relationships. Analyses of various items clarify these results. Hungarian adolescents' endorsement rate with respect to "I mostly enjoy getting together with friends" was consistently among the highest of the ten countries studied; 92% of Hungarian teenagers endorsed this item. Hungarian teenagers tended not to affirm that "when someone disagrees with me I get very mad." Only 15% of Hungarian teenagers endorsed this item.

The relatively poor social adjustment attested to by Bengali youths is illustrated by their high rate of endorsement of having difficulty making friends (31%) and being "very hurt or heartbroken if others do not agree with me" (62%). These endorsement rates are far higher than those manifested by youths of any other country studied. A result running contrary to the overall trend was that Bengali youths had the highest endorsement rate (62%) regarding not being upset if someone else corrects their mistakes, for they can learn from them.

Vocational and Educational Goals

Three countries showed consistent extreme scores with respect to vocational and educational goals. United States teenagers were consistently higher in this area, while teenagers from Israel and Hungary were consistently lower. One item in particular sharply differentiated the countries. This item concerned thinking about the kind of work the teenager will do in the future. United States teenagers affirmed this item at a relatively high rate (94%), while Israeli and Hungarian adolescents manifested somewhat lower rates of endorsement (85% and 87%, respectively). Clearly, however, the vast majority of teenagers in these countries nevertheless endorsed this item in a positive way. Another item that distinguished among the countries concerned feeling able to

TABLE 7. *Social Self: Items within Each Self Showing Consistent Intercountry Differences across Age and Gender*[a]

No.	Item	Australia	Bangladesh	Hungary	Israel	Italy	Taiwan	Turkey	United States	West Germany
					Percent endorsement					
37.	I am sure that I will be proud about my future profession.	83	78	68	87	76	66	89	90	78
58.	At times I think about what kind of work I will do in the future.	91	93	87	85	87	91	90	94	91
62.	I find it extremely hard to make friends.	16	31	16	19	22	22	25	11	11
65.	I do not mind being corrected, since I can learn from it.	84	96	82	72	69	88	61	83	79
79.	I feel that there is plenty I can learn from others.	87	90	88	80	91	94	89	94	84
86.	If others disapprove of me I get terribly upset.	43	62	15	21	28	42	43	39	33
124.	I enjoy most parties I go to.	88	85	92	78	69	51	75	87	83

[a] Items presented (1) were on a scale on which at least one country was consistently high (or low) in all four age-by-gender cells and (2) were consistently high (or low) for that country for that scale. Consistently high (or low) was defined in terms of being in the upper (or lower) third of nine countries in all four age-by-gender cells. Percentages shown are the average percent endorsement for that item for the country across four age-by-gender cells.

learn from others. While 80% of Israeli adolescents expressed feeling that they are able to learn from others, the endorsement of this item was even higher in the other countries. Further explicating differences among countries with respect to vocational and educational goals were the relatively low rates of endorsement shown by Hungarian youths with respect to the item "I am confident that I will be proud of my future vocation. Sixty-eight percent of Hungarian teenagers endorsed this item, the second lowest rate of all the countries studied.

Hungarian adolescents showed particularly interesting results with respect to the social self. They related more sociable, peer-oriented feelings. At the same time, they did not affirm high vocational and educational goals. The relatively poor social adjustment shown by Bengali youths parallels their psychological self-functioning. Perhaps Israeli teenagers' having relatively low investment in vocational and educational goals reflects the fact that most Israeli adolescents are going to go into the army, postponing vocational and educational careers. The more positive attitude toward vocational and educational goals shown by United States teenagers probably is associated with the greater range of opportunities with respect to both jobs and schools in this very wealthy country.

Sexual Self

Sexual Attitudes

With respect to sexual attitudes, two countries—Turkey and Taiwan—showed consistent extreme scores: Teenagers in these countries reported more conservative sexual attitudes (Table 8). These attitudes were revealed at the item level in this way: Turkish youths had a relatively low endorsement rate (19%) with respect to the item "Dirty jokes can sometimes be amusing." Turkish and Taiwanese youths were relatively high (22% and 27%, respectively) in their rate of affirming that thinking or talking about sex is frightening. One-third of Taiwanese youths, in addition, attested to feeling that "I am behind in sexual matters." This rate is higher than that shown by teenagers from any other country. Taiwanese adolescents tended to indicate that they do not feel the opposite sex finds them attractive (59%), do not feel that sexual experiences give them pleasure (78%), and do not feel that it is important to have "a good friend of the opposite sex" (48%). These rates also are higher than those manifested by teenagers from any other country.

These results indicate that attitudes toward sexuality among teenagers are very much culturally determined. In traditional societies such

TABLE 8. Sexual Self: Items within Each Self Showing Consistent Intercountry Differences across Age and Gender[a]

No.	Item	Australia	Bangladesh	Hungary	Israel	Italy	Taiwan	Turkey	United States	West Germany
						Percent endorsement				
28.	Dirty jokes are fun at times.	82	33	39	78	69	43	19	78	69
77.	I think that girls/boys find me attractive.	53	63	58	68	55	41	59	73	63
91.	Sexually I am way behind.	20	26	11	10	7	33	19	24	11
97.	Thinking or talking about sex scares me.	7	50	13	6	7	27	22	10	6
117.	Sexual experiences give me pleasure.	67	44	65	72	67	22	49	74	67
119.	Having a girl-/boyfriend is important to me.	69	77	68	75	76	52	74	73	82

[a] Items presented (1) were on a scale on which at least one country was consistently high (or low) in all four age-by-gender cells and (2) were consistently high (or low) for that country for that scale. Consistently high (or low) was defined in terms of being in the upper (or lower) third of nine countries in all four age-by-gender cells. Percentages shown are the average percent endorsement for that item for the country across four age-by-gender cells.

as Taiwan and Turkey, sex is both taboo and frightening to teenagers. In Taiwan, in particular, sexuality seems not to be comfortable or a priority for teenagers. Taiwanese youths not only tend to express feeling afraid of sex and being behind in sexual matters, they also tend to indicate that sexual experiences do not give them pleasure and that they do not feel it to be as important to have a good friend of the opposite sex as do teenagers in other countries.

Familial Self

Family Relationships

Israeli adolescents consistently reported more positive family relationships; Australian adolescents reported poorer family relationships (Table 9). These contrasts were reflected in the endorsement patterns of many individual items. About 90% of Israeli adolescents rated their parents as patient with them; in contrast, less than 70% of Australian teenagers affirmed their parents' patience. Israeli adolescents relatively rarely (9%) rated themselves as feeling that they are a bother or nuisance at home. Australian adolescents endorsed this item at a much higher rate (37%). Forty-six percent of the Australian teenagers—a much higher proportion than that shown by youths of any other country—expressed feeling that their parents are almost always on the side of someone else. Australian teenagers relatively frequently (39%) endorsed feeling that their parents do not understand a person because they had an unhappy childhood. In contrast, Israeli adolescents tended not to endorse loving "one of my parents much more than the other" (17%), or feeling that "my parents are ashamed of me" (3%). These endorsement rates are among the lowest for these items across the ten countries. The endorsement rate (41%) shown by Israeli youths with respect to one item—"When my parents are strict with me, I think they are right even if it angers me"—are unusually low and could be construed as running against the overall trend for Israeli youths to describe better family functioning. The very low endorsement rate of Israeli teenagers on one item was probably due to a mistranslation: In English the item in question read, "Very often I feel that my father is no good"; the Israeli endorsement rate for this item was 6%. When this item was back-translated from Hebrew to English it read, "I often feel like a failure." The relatively low level of endorsement of this item shown by Israeli teenagers may be an artifact of this mistranslation; at any rate, the mistranslation bars any interpretation of its significance.

The relatively good feelings related by Israeli adolescents about their families may reflect the traditional Jewish emphasis on family

TABLE 9. *Familial Self: Items within Each Self Showing Consistent Intercountry Differences across Age and Gender*[a]

No.	Item	Percent endorsement								
		Australia	Bangladesh	Hungary	Israel	Italy	Taiwan	Turkey	United States	West Germany
9.	My parents are almost always on the side of someone else, for example, my brother or sister.	46	35	24	22	21	21	20	29	13
21.	Very often I feel that my father is no good.	19	12	13	6	15	18	8	15	9
55.	When my parents are strict, I feel that they are right, even if I get angry.	61	86	64	41	68	75	71	61	38
71.	My parents are usually patient with me.	68	90	82	91	80	79	83	84	80
73.	Very often parents do not understand a person because they had an unhappy childhood.	39	21	24	20	28	15	34	25	34
85.	Usually I feel that I am a bother at home.	37	16	11	9	10	16	35	21	19
87.	I like one of my parents much better than the other.	26	39	19	17	20	40	24	28	27
95.	My parents are ashamed of me.	11	7	4	3	4	10	8	7	2
112.	Most of the time my parents are satisfied with me.	83	84	78	87	79	75	88	85	79

[a] Items presented (1) were on a scale on which at least one country was consistently high (or low) in all four age-by-gender cells and (2) were consistently high (or low) for that country for that scale. Consistently high (or low) was defined in terms of being in the upper (or lower) third of nine countries in all four age-by-gender cells. Percentages shown are the average percent endorsement for that item for the country across four age-by-gender cells.

relationships. Israeli adolescents clearly feel esteemed and appreciated by their parents. Even the Israeli youths' low endorsement of feeling their parents are right when they are strict could be interpreted as following the overall trend. It is possible that Israeli adolescents feel so esteemed by their parents that when there is a conflict with their parents they have the self-confidence to feel they are right and not their parents. The relatively poor family relationships reported by Australian adolescents seem to have no ready explanation.

Coping Self

Mastery of the External World

With respect to the Mastery of the External World scale, Israeli and United States adolescents consistently showed the most positive self-image, while Taiwanese youths consistently showed the most negative (Table 10). Using items to illustrate these trends: Israeli adolescents showed the highest endorsement (94%) level regarding feeling able to make decisions. Ninety-four percent of Israeli adolescents denied feeling that "I lack talent altogether." This rate of negation was the highest among the ten countries studied. Many (85%) United States adolescents denied feeling that "I find life an endless series of problems— without solution in sight." In contrast, 27% of Taiwanese teenagers indicated feeling that "I have no talent in any area." Taiwanese youths showed a relatively low level of endorsement (63%) when responding to the item "When I decide to do something, I do it."

Psychopathology

Four countries showed consistently extreme scale scores with respect to psychopathology. Data with respect to many items reflected these cross-national differences. German youths endorsed feeling confused at a relatively low level (9%); in contrast, Taiwanese and Bengali youths endorsed feeling confused (53% and 45%, respectively) at relatively high levels. Similarly, 75% of Hungarian and German youths tended to deny feeling guilty or blaming themselves when they had committed no wrong. Fifty-three and 54% of Taiwanese and Bengali youths indicated that they blame themselves needlessly. Eighty-eight percent of German and 81% of Hungarian youths denied feeling unable to get things done even though they are continuously on the go. Only 55% of Taiwanese youths denied this feeling. German youths' low level of psychopathology is illustrated by the fact that only 17% endorsed feeling so embarrassed that they feel like hiding in a corner and crying.

TABLE 10. Coping Self: Items within Each Self Showing Consistent Intercountry Differences across Age and Gender[a]

No.	Item	Percent endorsement								
		Australia	Bangladesh	Hungary	Israel	Italy	Taiwan	Turkey	United States	West Germany
2.	When I am with people, I am afraid that someone will make fun of me.	26	29	10	21	29	35	36	23	13
22.	I am confused most of the time.	19	45	31	12	21	53	47	17	9
29.	I often blame myself even when I am not at fault.	40	46	25	26	40	47	34	36	25
31.	The size of my sex organs is normal.	91	87	90	94	97	86	76	91	98
36.	Sometimes I feel so ashamed of myself that I just want to hide in a corner and cry.	30	31	20	25	22	32	24	25	17
45.	I feel empty emotionally most of the time.	27	39	12	20	29	47	42	18	8
49.	Our society is a competitive one and I am not afraid of it.	64	85	60	65	46	69	67	72	49
53.	I find it very difficult to establish new friendships.	24	42	25	25	26	27	32	21	23
56.	Working closely with another fellow never gives me pleasure.	29	22	19	26	19	14	32	28	14
61.	I often feel that I would rather die than go on living.	30	38	17	19	15	14	25	19	19
76.	When I decide to do something, I do it.	77	82	84	84	74	63	87	86	83
84.	If I know that I will have to face a new situation, I will try in advance to find out as much as is possible about it.	79	92	87	80	87	91	86	85	86
93.	Even though I am continuously on the go, I seem unable to get things done.	33	42	19	24	21	45	35	32	12
96.	I believe I can tell the real from the fantastic.	71	63	87	90	72	84	84	85	84
103.	I find life an endless series of problems—without solution in sight.	27	39	11	23	13	31	37	15	18
105.	I feel that I am able to make decisions.	81	88	86	94	78	77	78	90	90
109.	I feel that I have no talent whatsoever.	15	22	9	6	32	27	17	10	8
110.	I do not rehearse how I might deal with a real coming event.	43	39	28	44	25	25	35	34	37
114.	I do not enjoy solving difficult problems.	43	24	45	36	44	25	43	36	24
121.	Worrying a little about one's future helps to make it work out better.	62	90	79	75	84	89	79	69	82

[a] Items presented (1) were on a scale on which at least one country was consistently high (or low) in all four age-by-gender cells and (2) were consistently high (or low) for that country for that scale. Consistently high (or low) was defined in terms of being in the upper (or lower) third of nine countries in all four age-by-gender cells. Percentages shown are the average percent endorsement for that item for the country across four age-by-gender cells.

This rate of endorsement was the lowest across all ten countries. In contrast, 38% of Bengali adolescents reported that they would rather be dead than alive. This rate of endorsement was the highest across all ten countries. Running against the overall trend, Taiwanese youths showed a relatively low endorsement rate (14%) with respect to preferring to be dead to being alive.

It is important to remember that results with respect to several items on this scale may be an artifact of poor translations. The apparent relatively high level of psychopathology shown by Bengali youths is not confirmed by their low level of endorsement of an item that in the original read, "I believe I can tell the real from the fantastic." A low level of endorsement for the original item might indicate psychopathology, but low endorsements corresponding to the Bengali back-translation—"I believe that I can give something imagined the form of a true story"—do not necessarily indicate high levels of psychopathology. Similarly, German and Hungarian youths were relatively unlikely to report feeling emotionally empty; Taiwanese and Bengali adolescents endorsed this item at relatively high levels. But the Taiwanese and Bengali back-translations indicate that the meaning of the original item may not have been preserved. The back-translation from the Chinese was "I often feel empty"; the back-translation from the Bengali was "Mentally, most of the time, I feel empty of emotions." Since feeling empty might not refer to emotional emptiness and the meaning of "mentally feeling empty of emotions" is not clear, these back-translations may not have preserved the original meaning of the item, and the corresponding endorsement rates may not be meaningful.

Superior Adjustment

Bengali and Taiwanese youths' scale scores indicated relatively high levels of adjustment in this area; Australian youths' scale scores indicated relatively low levels of adjustment in this area. Bengali and Taiwanese youths' good adjustment in this area is reflected by the fact that 92% and 91%, respectively, endorse the item "If I know that I will have to encounter a new situation then I try to find out about it in advance." These endorsement rates are the highest across the ten countries. In contrast, Australian youths endorsed this item at a relatively low level (79%). Taiwanese and Bengali teenagers tended to assert that worrying about one's future helps make it work out better. Their endorsement rates—89% and 90%—were the highest among the countries studied for this item. Relatively few (25% and 24%, respectively) Taiwanese and Bengali adolescents indicated they did not like solving difficult problems. Eighty-five percent of Bengali youths affirmed believing that while society is competitive, they are not frightened of it, the highest rate across countries for this item. Taiwanese adolescents rarely affirmed (14%) that working closely with other people has never given them pleasure. One item seemed to reflect a trend contrary to the scale scores: Bengali youths, who generally reported very good adjustment in this area, affirmed at a relatively high level (42%) finding it difficult to establish new friendships. This rate was the highest for this item across the countries studied.

Overall, with respect to the coping self, Israeli and United States adolescents showed the most positive attitudes. In accord with comments made in the familial self section, results suggest that Israeli adolescents are confident, perhaps owing to the investment of their parents in them. Thus, Israeli adolescents tend to feel able to make decisions and not to feel they lack talent. A relatively high proportion of United States adolescents expressed confidence about the future. The picture presented by Taiwanese teenagers is more complicated. Many express low confidence with respect to having talent and with respect to decision making. Many Taiwanese teenagers reported feeling confused and unable to make a decision. In contrast, Taiwanese youths tended not to affirm preferring to be dead to being alive. They tended to endorse planning for the future and needing to prepare beforehand. Similarly, a relatively large proportion of Bengali teenagers affirmed that they would rather be dead than alive. Many stated that they tend to blame themselves needlessly. Yet a relatively large percentage of Bengali youths endorsed trying to find out about a new situation in advance; they tended to relate that while society is competitive, they are not afraid of it. German adolescents tended to show relatively good functioning in this area. A relatively high proportion reported not feeling confused and not blaming themselves when they had committed no wrong. They tended to deny feeling unable to accomplish anything and tended not to affirm feeling a great deal of embarrassment. Just as they tended to affirm poor family functioning, Australian youths showed relatively high rates of endorsement of poor coping. Planning for the future or trying to find out about new situations in advance seems to be a problem area for many Australian youths sampled here.

Individual Values

Five of the six items that were not included on any scale (see Table 11) showed consistent cross-national difference. As can be seen, these items are concerned with values. Results show that Italian teenagers affirmed not wanting to hurt someone just for the "heck of it" at a relatively high rate (78%); in contrast, Hungarian teenagers were rela-

TABLE 11. Individual Values: Items Showing Consistent Intercountry Differences across Age and Gender[a]

No.	Item				Percent endorsement					
		Australia	Bangladesh	Hungary	Israel	Italy	Taiwan	Turkey	United States	West Germany
5.	I would not hurt someone just for the "heck of it."	74	64	64	72	78	66	86	81	67
40.	I blame others even when I know that I am at fault too.	35	25	11	22	38	27	11	29	13
48.	Telling the truth means nothing to me.	20	23	11	14	18	16	6	10	20
67.	I do not care how my actions affect others as long as I gain something.	21	22	16	27	10	12	30	11	12
120.	I would not like to be associated with those kids who "hit below the belt."	63	82	81	73	74	88	78	71	77

[a] Items presented (1) were on a scale on which at least one country was consistently high (or low) in all four age-by-gender cells and (2) were consistently high (or low) for that country for that scale. Consistently high (or low) was defined in terms of being in the upper (or lower) third of nine countries in all four age-by-gender cells. Percentages shown are the average percent endorsement for that item for the country across four age-by-gender cells.

tively low (64%) in their denying not wanting to hurt someone just for the "heck of it." Turkish teenagers affirmed not wanting to hurt someone at a relatively high rate (86%), but that rate may have been a function of a mistranslation since the Turkish back-translation for this item was "I would not offend anyone by saying 'I don't care.'" Hungarian and German teenagers tended not to endorse (11% and 13%, respectively) "I blame others even when I know that I am at fault too." Australian and Italian teenagers did tend to affirm blaming others (35% and 38%). Israeli and Turkish teenagers manifested relatively high rates of endorsement (27% and 30%), while Italian teenagers showed relatively low rates of endorsement (10%) regarding the item "I do not care how my actions affect others as long as I gain something." Eighty-eight percent of Taiwanese youths asserted they did not want to be associated with kids who "hit below the belt"; only 63% of Australian youths affirmed this item.

Moral attitudes were not the monopoly of teenagers from any single country. Results with respect to some countries were somewhat contradictory. Thus, Italian teenagers affirmed not wanting to hurt someone "just for the heck of it." At the same time they affirmed blaming others even when they know they are at fault too. Hungarian teenagers showed a different pattern, with many asserting wanting to hurt someone "just for the heck of it," and relatively few affirming blaming others even when they know they are at fault too. Italian teenagers denied not caring how their actions affect others as long as they can gain something. The relative self-confidence of Israeli teenagers may find its counterpart in their relatively high endorsement of not caring how their actions affect others as long as they can gain something.

Conclusion

In no instance were adolescents from one country better off or better adjusted in *all* areas than adolescents from all other countries. There were strengths and weaknesses of adolescent functioning in every country we studied.

DEPRESSION OR QUIET DISTURBANCE AMONG ADOLESCENTS

Adolescents throughout the world, our data show, have a positive self-image. But that fact does not preclude recognizing a darker side: that in all countries there is a substantial minority of adolescents who have a difficult time coping and who have a poor self-image. We now turn our attention to a salient emotional issue that confronts the teenagers of our time—depression, sometimes manifested as "quiet disturbance"—emotional disturbance that is not shown through acting-out behavior or other highly visible symptomatology (Ostrov, 1986). Relevant to this group, findings of epidemiological studies have been remarkably consistent: In various nations, among disparate groups, about 20% of adolescents manifest significant emotional disturbance (Graham and Rutter, 1973; Kandel and Davies, 1982; Krupinski et al., 1967; Langner, Gersten, and Eisenberg, 1974; Rutter, Graham, Chadwick, and Yule, 1976). Many are socially alienated during a life-stage that involves consolidation of identity, changing relationships with adults, and socialization through peer relationships. They experience depression and a lowered self-esteem that may persist throughout life as an adult. As a context for this finding, however, it is important to note that the rate of depression among adolescents is about the same as that found among older age groups.

In this section we shall first review the literature describing depression and quiet disturbance among teenagers. Contrasts between the prevalence of these conditions among teenage boys as compared to teenage girls will be emphasized. Lastly, results showing the incidence of depression and alienation among the adolescents that we studied will be presented.

Rates of Psychological Disturbance

Findings regarding adolescents can best be appreciated in the context of results of recent epidemiological surveys of the U.S. adult population. Mellinger et al. (1978) conducted a national household survey and found that "27% of American adults experienced high levels of psychic distress during the year prior to interview" (p. 1047). They reported that "psychic distress" was more prevalent among women than among men. Thirty-four percent of the women were classified as high on psychic distress as compared with 19% of the men. Reviewing 12 studies, Boyd and Weissman (1981) concluded that 9 to 20% of the population have depressive symptoms at any one time (point prevalence). They also found that rates were higher for women than for men. Meyers et al. (1984) reported that the median point prevalence rate of psychiatric disorders across three sites was 20%. Epidemiological research on mental illness among adults in the Western world has consistently shown a rate hovering around 20% (Freedman, 1984; Offer and Spiro, 1987).

In light of the "turmoil" theories of adolescence (e.g., Blos, 1961;

A. Freud, 1958; Rabichow and Sklansky, 1980), it might be expected
that the prevalence of psychiatric symptoms would be higher among
teenagers than among adults. Yet data stemming from studies of adolescents do not support that conclusion. Instead, prevalence rates of psychiatric disturbance among teenagers are very similar to those found
among adults. Krupinski et al. (1967) conducted an epidemiological
study of teenagers in the small Australian town of Heyfield. They concluded that 16% of the male adolescents and 19% of the female adolescents in the town had psychiatrically diagnosable conditions. A Scandinavian study (Bjornsson, 1974) of 13- to 14-year-old adolescents in an
industrial town reported the prevalence of moderate or severe psychiatric disorder to be 21% for boys and 14% for girls.

A series of studies by Rutter and his colleagues (Graham and Rutter, 1973; Rutter et al., 1976) were conducted on the Isle of Wight, an
island off the coast of England containing small towns and villages.
Information was based on psychiatric interviews of the youths and
their parents and teachers. According to the authors, "more than a fifth
of the boys and girls reported that they felt miserable or depressed, and
the same proportion reported great difficulty in sleeping and waking
unnecessarily early in the morning" (Rutter et al., 1976, p. 42). Using
parents' interviews as the source of information about adolescents,
these researchers found that the prevalence of psychiatric disorder
among 14-year-olds was 13%. After compiling figures from multiple
data sources, it was concluded that "the corrected prevalence rate for
psychiatric disorder in 14- to 15-year-old children was 21%" (Graham
and Rutter, p. 1227).

Relatively few studies of the prevalence and kind of emotional
disturbance among adolescents have been conducted in the United
States. This has remained true even though eight years have elapsed
since Locksley and Douvan (1979) wrote, "Although national [United
States] surveys of the incidence of psychopathology among adolescents
have not been conducted as yet, this may be a direction for research
ultimately as profitable as those directions heretofore pursued" (p. 73).

Langner et al. (1974) used a questionnaire administered to mothers
regarding their children's behavior to study the epidemiology of U.S.
adolescent psychiatric illness. Their sample consisted of 1,034 children aged 6 to 18 who were randomly selected within a cross-section of
Manhattan in New York City. Questionnaire results were rated by a
psychiatrist for degree of impairment. Findings were that 17 to 20% of
the black and Spanish children studied displayed extreme rates of impairment, while only 8 to 9% of the white children showed these extreme rates. Unfortunately, results were not reported separately for adolescents. Studying small samples of seventh- and eighth-graders from

one parochial school in suburban Philadelphia, and using the Beck Depression Inventory as a source of data, Albert and Beck (1975) found that 31.3% of their early adolescent sample fell into the range of moderate to severe depressive symptomatology, while another 2.2% fell into the severe range.

Kandel and Davies (1982) studied the epidemiology of depression among adolescents 14 to 18 years of age who were representative of public high school students in New York State in 1971 and 1972. They found that adolescents from families with very low incomes were more depressed than were those from any other socioeconomic-status group. Girls were more depressed than were boys. The one prevalence rate cited in this study indicated that 20% of the adolescents reported "feeling sad or depressed in the past year."

Recently, we conducted a study in the Chicago area (Offer, Ostrov, and Howard, 1987) to learn more about emotional disturbance and mental health resource utilization among adolescents. Results indicated that about 20% of the adolescents studied were psychologically disturbed. It should be noted that many of these troubled youngsters were "quietly disturbed"—that is, they had never been seen by a mental health professional, they had never come to the attention of the authorities, nor had they been perceived by adults as needing help.

Turning to gender differences in rate of depression, most studies indicate that teenage boys and girls do not differ with respect to global self-esteem. But studies that consider various dimensions of self-esteem generally show that (1) girls view themselves more positively than do boys with regard to interpersonal relationships and sociability (Helland, 1973; Monge, 1973; Wiggins, 1973), while (2) boys view themselves more positively than do girls with regard to achievement (Monge, 1973), academic aspirations (Wiggins, 1973), self-assertion (Gregory, 1977), and body image (Clifford, 1971; Healey and Deblassie, 1974; Musa and Roach, 1973). Offer, Ostrov, and Howard (1981a) reported that, in a large national sample, adolescent boys attested to less depression, less neurotic adjustment, and better body image than did adolescent girls.

Another study (Offer, Ostrov, and Howard, 1984) used two cohorts of teenagers, one studied four years earlier than the other, to learn about nonhistorical period-dependent boy–girl self-image differences. Consistent gender effects were found across the four-year period for both younger and older teenagers: Boys reported better impulse control, less depression, and better body image than did the girls. To explicate these findings: 72 to 78% of boys (percents are given separately for younger [13- to 15-year-old] and older [16- to 19-year-old] groups, respectively) reported being able to remain calm under pressure, while only 64 to

70% of the girls did so. Among boys, 13 to 17% attested to being very lonely, while 22 to 40% of the girls did so. Feeling ugly and unattractive was endorsed by 16 to 26% of the boys and 38 to 55% of the girls. Being confused most of the time was endorsed by 9 to 17% of the boys and 20 to 25% of the girls. Only 15 to 21% of the boys attested to at times feeling "so ashamed of myself I just want to hide in a corner and cry"; 26 to 52% of the girls endorsed this item.

These findings suggest that depression, at least among American teenagers, is more likely to occur among girls than among boys. When girls are disturbed they may be more prone to *quiet* disturbance than are disturbed boys, because girls are less likely to act out negative feelings. Conversely, since acting out negative feelings is more usual among boys, boys who are quietly disturbed may be more psychiatrically ill than girls who are quietly disturbed. Findings presented in Offer et al. (1987) confirm the higher incidence of quiet disturbance among girls and the greater pathology of quietly disturbed boys.

That learning more about depressed adolescents is important is indicated by recent findings about suicide among adolescents. Almost all the data available to us are from the United States. At times persons concerned about suicide among teenagers lose sight of the fact that at their highest, the rate of suicides among U.S. teenagers does not exceed 12 per 100,000 (so that the odds are against one suicide in any one year in a high school of 5,000). The suicide rate among U.S. teenagers is lower than that for almost all other age groups in the U.S., especially elderly people. The suicide rate for U.S. teenagers has leveled off in recent years, apparently as a function of the declining proportion of adolescents within the total U.S. population (Holinger and Offer, 1982). On the other side of the coin, as Peck (1982) wrote, "In the late 1960s, the suicide rate among young people began increasing . . . from the years 1961 through 1975, suicide rates among 15- to 24-year-olds increased 131% while the suicide rate of the population as a whole increased only 22%" (pp. 29–30). According to Crumley (1982), "the rate [of suicide for 15- to 19-year-olds] has actually doubled from 1968 to 1976. Approximately 5,000 deaths per year are now attributed to suicide among teenagers" (p. 158).

Regarding teenagers who commit suicide, Peck (1981) wrote that a substantial number of suicides occur in a group composed primarily of young white males who appear to be isolated in their life-style and relationships. It is from this group of suicidal youngsters that he identified "the loner." According to Crumley (1982), feelings of abandonment, loneliness, and isolation are prominent among adolescents who attempt suicide. Diagnostically, Crumley (1982) states that among suicidal adolescents, depressive syndromes are by far the most common.

Hudgens (1974) reported that 31% of adolescents hospitalized with a history of attempted suicide made that attempt without having any psychiatric care and without telling about the attempt until much later. On the basis of his clinical experience with suicidal adolescents, Tabachnick (1981) wrote:

> Suicidal people often describe a feeling of loneliness, or a sense of being alienated from the whole world . . . associated with the suicidal states are episodes of hopelessness. . . . Often a lack of hope is associated with an inner feeling of emptiness. (p. 401)

Schrut (1964) concluded that progressive or continued isolation in early childhood is indicative of a more serious prognosis for suicide than an early history that indicates an ability to form interpersonal relationships.

Similarly, Farberow (1983) found that suicide among teenagers was related to depression, withdrawal, and interpersonal isolation, among other factors. Surveying adolescent suicide attempt statistics, Marks and Haller (1977, p. 391) noted, "It becomes obvious that many adolescent suicide attempts go unnoticed, or at least unreported." On the basis of their large study sample of adolescent psychiatric patients, Marks and Haller (1977) showed that as compared with non-suicide attempters, adolescents referred for suicide attempts are characterized by sadness, emotionality, and a proclivity to react to frustration intropunitively. Male suicide attempters were described as continuing to lack close relationships with male peers. Female suicide attempters were described as characteristically having few or no friends during childhood and not being able to talk about their personal problems with anyone. During adolescence, female suicide attempters were described as seldom attending church, not valuing friendships, and continuing to feel alienated from their fathers. Marks and Haller (1977, p. 339) concluded, "Our sample of suicidal adolescent girls do indeed have histories of social isolation coupled with feelings of parental rejection."

Indicative, too, of the importance of studying depressed adolescents are studies showing the persistence of emotional disturbance during the teenage years into adulthood. As Mitchell (1980) put it (p. 200), "Studies . . . show that many disturbed adolescents do not 'grow out of it,' as had previously been believed." To illustrate these studies, Vaillant and McArthur (1972) found that even among subjects initially selected for good adjustment, moderately high correlations pertain between an index of adjustment during adolescence and an index of adjustment during middle-age years. That correlation is more impressive because it would tend to be greatly decreased, owing to the restriction on range of adjustment caused by the high selectivity of the subjects studied. Masterson (1967) followed a group of adolescent psychiatric patients for five years and found that they remained more disturbed than did controls throughout the follow-up period. Weiner and DelGaudio (1976) found that many of the adolescent psychiatric patients they followed were readmitted for psychiatric illnesses as adults. Doane, West, Goldstein, Rodnick, and Jones (1981) accurately predicted that many adolescents referred for treatment would become schizophrenic as young adults or manifest other serious psychiatric illnesses. Offer et al. (1984) found that about 50% of disturbed teenagers—as shown by their having a negative self-image in a number of areas—remained disturbed when studied a year and a half later.

It was toward exploring the prevalence of depression among teenagers—and in particular toward exploring gender differences in the prevalence of depression among teenagers—in a cross-national context that the data analysis described in this chapter was undertaken. The prevalence of quiet disturbance will have to remain a matter for speculation since no data regarding acting out or recognition of disturbance by others were available.

Data Analysis

Details concerning construction of the Depression Scale were presented in the Method section. To briefly restate what was described there, we reviewed the items composing the International OSIQ and selected five (5) that represented depression, loneliness, or emotional emptiness. A Depression scale was composed using these five items. Adequate reliability of this scale was demonstrated. A depressed adolescent was defined as a youth whose average item endorsement showed sadness, loneliness, and emptiness. Rates of depression were calculated for each gender-by-age group for each of the ten countries.

The five items included in the scale are listed in Table 12.

Results

Table 13 shows the percent of teenagers who scored in the depressed range on this scale. Average rates of depression across countries ranged from 14 to 48%. Bengali and Japanese teenagers consistently ranked as the most depressed among the ten countries studied. West German teenagers were least depressed on the average. Among younger teenagers, Hungarian youths ranked as the least depressed. Considering age and gender cells across countries, at least 10% of the adolescents in

TABLE 12. Depression

Item no.	English version of the item[a]
45.	I feel empty emotionally most of the time.
61.	I often feel that I would rather die than go on living.
66.	I feel so very lonely.
103.	I find life an endless series of problems—without solution in sight.
130.	I frequently feel sad.

[a] Back-translations of the items can be found in Appendix 1.

any cell were depressed. Overall, 27% of teenagers reported feeling depressed.

For all ten countries, extent of depression among males and females was compared separately for younger and older teenagers. Nineteen comparisons were made (only older teenagers were available for the Japanese comparison). Of these 19 comparisons, 17 showed more depression among females. A similar comparison between older and younger teenagers across males and females for the nine countries (excluding Japan) produced results that were not consistent in direction across countries.

These results indicate that a significant minority of adolescents in countries throughout the world are depressed. Taking the lowest per-

TABLE 13. Percent Endorsement for the Five Items Constituting the Depression Scale[a]

Country	Younger males	Older males	Younger females	Older females	Mean
Australia	27	23	35	34	30
Bangladesh	42	42	52	56	48
Hungary	10	18	12	19	15
Israel	17	19	18	29	21
Italy	15	18	34	23	22
Japan	—	45	—	44	44
Taiwan	23	38	27	38	31
Turkey	33	37	33	42	36
United States	16	18	25	20	20
West Germany	17	11	17	11	14
Average	22	27	28	32	27

[a] Percentages have been rounded to the nearest whole number.

cent found—10%—and considering that the adolescents constitute approximately 10% of the total population of the world, results indicate that there are about 60 million depressed teenagers.

These findings raise a number of developmental, epidemiological, and methodological issues. Developmentally, the data suggest that adolescents are no more filled with turmoil or emotional disturbance than are persons at any other stage of life—at least not in those countries for which we have adult-relevant data. The overall figure of 27% does not differ markedly from the 20% figure found cross-culturally among adults (Freedman, 1984; Offer and Spiro, 1987). This finding does not imply that disturbance may not be qualitatively different in adolescence. Disturbance during adolescence may have special emotional qualities—a sense of having let life pass by may be less prevalent, for instance; body image problems may be more prevalent. But the extent of disturbance does not seem different. As has been the case with respect to almost every empirical study of teenagers, these results cast a heavy shadow of doubt upon those developmental theories that describe unusual and especially marked disturbance among adolescents.

From an epidemiological perspective, it is notable that in studies in the United States we found that about 50% of the adolescents who need mental health care do not get help (Offer et al., 1987). Only one-quarter of the disturbed group, or about 5% of the total adolescent population, obtained extended mental health care, defined as at least three mental health visits. It is likely that in less developed countries, a still smaller percent receive treatment. The implication is that there are many millions of adolescents in need of treatment who are not receiving help.

From a cross-cultural view, the high rate of depression among Bengali youths may reflect the great poverty of and difficult living conditions within that country. There are conditions that adolescents, or persons of any age, cannot adjust to—extreme poverty and deprivation is disturbing and depressing, and those of our adolescent subjects in that condition express it. The reason for the relatively high rate of depression among Japanese youths is less clear. The pressure for achievement placed upon teenagers in that country may exact a high toll at a feeling level.

The greater depression of girls appears consistent with our findings in this Chapter. Cross-culturally, teenage girls appear to be at greater risk of depression than are teenage boys. Yet they may not show that depression or receive help because of their more sociable and less aggressive stance. This point should be understood in the context of findings (Offer, Ostrov, and Howard, 1986b) indicating that quietly disturbed adolescents will respond positively if helping professionals or other adults reach out to them. Reaching out to disturbed girls may be particularly important in terms of reaching large numbers of hitherto unhelped emotionally troubled adolescents.

Almost nothing is known about the developmental course of depressed adolescents who do not receive psychiatric help during their teenage years. Given the persistence of adjustment across the life-span, though, it seems unlikely that depressed adolescents simply "grow out of it." Many may grow up to be disturbed adults, perhaps in some cases transmitting their unhappiness to a subsequent generation of adolescents. They may never reach out for or receive necessary psychiatric help or counseling.

For many depressed adolescents, it may be necessary to reach out to give help. It may be necessary to offer help in an innovative way and to be sensitive to *sub rosa* pleas for help and to ask whether help is needed. Offering a helping relationship to depressed adolescents might yield a surprisingly receptive response in return. It also might save a great deal of suffering in the long run.

DEMOGRAPHY, THE ECONOMY, AND ADOLESCENT SELF-IMAGE

The primary focus of this book is on characteristics held in common by the vast majority of adolescents in ten countries. We also explored contrasts among groups of adolescents. To this point we have discussed self-image differences between younger and older and between male and female teenagers. In this section we explore the potential influence of socioeconomic and demographic variables on various aspects of adolescent self-image.

In recent years there has been increasing interest in the impact of socioeconomic and demographic variables on social phenomena. Studies have described the influence of these variables on the rate and prevalence of physical illness (e.g., Brenner, 1979), self-destructive behavior (e.g., Holinger and Offer, 1982; Holinger, Offer, and Ostrov, 1987), and other social problems (e.g., Easterlin, 1980). There has always been considerable theoretical interest in deciphering the relationships between sociodemographic and psychological variables, but it has not been until newer, faster, and more efficient ways of researching both fields have evolved that this type of undertaking has been made possible.

In order to explore the relationship between these kinds of information, we selected available socioeconomic and demographic variables from data available to us from the United Nations (1985) as well as from individual contacts with the diplomatic missions of the nine countries in the United States.* The 18 variables selected had two things in common: (1) They were available from all of the countries, and (2) it made theoretical sense to include them, in light of past studies (e.g., Brenner, 1979; Easterlin, 1980; Holinger and Offer, 1982; Holinger et al., 1987).

Countries in each of the four age-by-gender groups (younger males, younger females, older males, and older females) were rank-ordered on the basis of each of their mean OSIQ scale scores. As a result, four sets of ranks were generated for each of the ten OSIQ scales. Similarly, the countries were rank-ordered with respect to each of the 18 economic and demographic variables. Rank-order correlations ($N = 9$; Japan was not included because younger age groups were not available for that country) were calculated between each OSIQ scale and each demographic variable for each of the four age-by-gender groups. An association between a scale score and an economic or demographic variable was interpreted if all four correlations were in the same direction and at least three of the four correlations between that scale score and that variable were statistically significant ($p < .05$). Since the four age-by-gender groups represent independent samples for each country, obtaining significance in at least three groups represents an extremely low probability of any finding's having occurred by chance alone (less than 1 chance in 10,000). Setting the probability of chance findings so low makes spurious findings unlikely, despite the fact that the significance of many correlations between OSIQ variables and economic/ demographic variables was tested.

Results

Six demographic/economic variables met the criteria for significant association with at least one OSIQ scale; 12 did not. The 6 variables that did meet our statistical criteria were these:

1. Gross national product
2. Per capita income
3. Physical quality of life index (a composite of statistics concerning infant mortality, life expectancy, and literacy)
4. Percent of 14- to 18-year-olds in the total population
5. Educational expenditure per capita
6. Percent of 15- to 19-year-old males in the labor force

---

*We are grateful to all the nine diplomatic missions, whose help was essential and who were always cordial and eager to cooperate.

These variables were consistently and significantly correlated with various OSIQ scales. They will be discussed in detail. The other 12 variables did not yield significant relationships. The variables studied that were not consistently significantly correlated with OSIQ scales were as follows:

1. Population density
2. Percent of population living in urban areas
3. Index of net social progress
4. Number of television sets per 1,000 individuals
5. Percent of gross national product spent on education
6. Percent of students enrolled in secondary schools
7. Postsecondary-school enrollment per 1,000 students
8. Percent of 15- to 19-year-old females in the labor force
9. Marriage rate among 15- to 19-year-old females
10. Marriage rate among 15- to 19-year-old males
11. Birth rate among 15- to 19-year-old mothers
12. Divorce rate of 15- to 19-year-olds

With regard to the OSIQ, the following four scales did not consistently correlate with any demographic and/or economic variable: Impulse Control, Family Relationships, Vocational and Educational Goals, and Superior Adjustment. The six other OSIQ scales did consistently and significantly correlate with demographic and economic variables (see Tables 14 through 19).

As shown in Table 14, adolescents' emotional tone, or mood, was positively related to their country's relative gross national product (GNP). In all four age-by-gender groups, the higher a country's economic output (and presumably the greater a country's wealth), the more positive the affect reported by its teenagers. Another significant correlation indicated that the higher the proportion of adolescents in a country's population, the less positive the affect reported by its teenagers. Adolescents' mood apparently is a function of their country's

TABLE 14. OSIQ Scale: Emotional Tone

	Younger males	Older males	Younger females	Older females
Gross National Product (GNP)	.65[a]	.67[a]	.68[a]	.79[a]
Percent of 14- to 18-year-olds in the total population	−.79[a]	−.80[a]	−.64[a]	−.74[a]

[a] Significant at the $p < .05$ level (two-tailed test; 7 df).

TABLE 15. OSIQ Scale: Body and Self-Image

	Younger males	Older males	Younger females	Older females
Per capita income	.78[a]	.80[a]	.52	.68[a]

[a] Significant at the $p < .05$ level (two-tailed test; 7 df).

relative wealth. The wealthier the country, the better the adolescents' mood. On the other hand, the more adolescents per capita, the worse a country's adolescents' mood.

Adolescents' body image (see Table 15) was correlated with only one demographic/economic variable: per capita income. The higher a country's per capita income, the more positive its adolescents felt about their bodies and health. Body image, in short, appears to be a function of wealth available for individuals in contrast to mood, which seems to be more responsive to a nation's total wealth. Perhaps for adolescents, high income at the individual level is linked primarily with having the time, resources, and incentive to achieve good health, physical fitness, and the accoutrements that facilitate good body image.

The Social Relationships scale (Table 16) was related to more demographic and economic variables than was any other OSIQ scale. Like emotional tone, social relationships was related in a positive way to GNP and in a negative way to percent of 14- to 18-year-olds in the total population. Social relationships also was related to two other demographic/economic variables. Good social (or peer) relationships was associated with (1) higher educational expenditures per capita and (2) a more positive physical quality of life. It is possible that among the areas of functioning tapped by the OSIQ, relationships with peers is most

TABLE 16. OSIQ Scale: Social Relationships

	Younger males	Older males	Younger females	Older females
Gross National Product (GNP)	.70[a]	.60[a]	.47	.82[a]
Percent of 14- to 18-year-olds in the total population	−.84[a]	−.76[a]	−.59[a]	−.74[a]
Educational expenditures per capita	.63[a]	.64[a]	.52	.83[a]
Quality of life index[b]	.59[a]	.69[a]	.38	.67[a]

[a] Significant at the $p < .05$ level (two-tailed test; 7 df).
[b] Based on literacy, life expectancy, and infant mortality.

TABLE 17. OSIQ Scale: Sexual Attitudes

	Younger males	Older males	Younger females	Older females
Per capita income	.35	.58^a	.75^a	.87^a
Quality of life index^b	.54	.79^a	.70^a	.77^a

^{a} Significant at the $p < .05$ level (two-tailed test; 7 df).
^{b} Based on literacy, life expectancy, and infant mortality.

affected by the economic resources available for, and the demographic variables impinging upon, teenagers. Very positive peer relationships seem to be a luxury of relatively well-advantaged adolescents.

A high score on the Sexual Attitudes scale (Table 17) represents liberal sexual attitudes. Liberal sexual attitudes were linked with a country's having a relatively high per capita income. In addition, a country's having a good quality of life was connected with that country's adolescents' having liberal sexual attitudes.

Mastery of the external world is a measure of adolescents' perceptions regarding their ability to cope with external challenges. Table 18 shows that in countries where adolescents constitute a low percentage of the total labor force, teenagers reported relatively good ability to cope. The better coping of adolescents in countries in which they form a relatively low proportion of the labor force may be a function of adolescents' reference or comparison groups. Adolescents in the work force or about to enter it may be comparing themselves unfavorably to older persons already working. Adolescents who do not face the necessity of work compare themselves to each other; presumably, compared to other adolescents it is relatively easy for teenagers to conclude they are competent.

A high score on the Psychopathology scale is indicative of low incidence of emotional symptoms (such as anxiety or loneliness). Table 19 shows a significant relationship between psychopathology and two

TABLE 18. OSIQ Scale: Mastery of the External World

	Younger males	Older males	Younger females	Older females
Percent of 15- to 19-year-old males in the labor force	−.83^a	−.12	−.67^a	−.72^a

^{a} Significant at the $p < .05$ level (two-tailed test; 7 df).

TABLE 19. OSIQ Scale: Psychopathology

	Younger males	Older males	Younger females	Older females
Percent of 14- to 18-year-olds in the total population	$-.76^a$	$-.72^a$	$-.72^a$	$-.74^a$
Education expenditure per capita	.53	$.62^a$	$.62^a$	$.65^a$

[a] Significant at the $p < .05$ level (two-tailed test; 7 df).

economic/demographic variables. A high proportion of 14- to 18-year-olds in the total population was associated with more manifest psychopathology. The other association adduced by these data was that the more money spent per capita by a country on education, the lower the reported psychopathology.

The economic/demographic variable most highly associated with aspects of adolescent self-image was the proportion of adolescents in the total population of a particular country. A high proportion of adolescents in a country's population was associated with adolescents' reporting relatively poor mood, poorer social relationships, and higher psychopathology. This association is consistent with the work of Easterlin (1980), Hendin (1982), Holinger and Offer (1982), and Holinger et al. (1987).

Perhaps surprisingly, gross national product (GNP) was more highly associated with self-image than was per capita income. Per capita income might be thought to be more related to an individual's quality of life than is GNP, which is summed across all individuals in the country no matter what their number. In fact, higher GNP was associated with both good emotional tone and positive peer relationships, while higher per capita income was associated only with better body image. This relationship may reflect the relatively good quality of life that a higher GNP may bring. But in addition, it may reflect identification by individual teenagers with a relatively powerful and wealthy entity—their country—an influence apart from any individual economic benefit. Quality of life, a variable that is broader than just income or wealth, was correlated with good social relationships and liberal sexual attitudes, again underlining the influence of economic/demographic advantage on peer relations.

Perhaps as interesting as knowing which OSIQ scales correlated with economic/demographic variables is considering which did not. Adolescents' family relationships and commitments, as we have seen, tend to be strong no matter what the economics or demographics of the country they are living in. Teenagers from all the countries studied tended to have positive vocational and educational goals. There was a roughly equal degree of affirmation of good impulse control across all the countries providing data. Adolescents' belief in their ability to learn to cope (superior adjustment) did not vary significantly by the wealth, resources, or economic/demographic practices of the country in which they lived.

We are aware of the fact that our attempt to correlate what is, on the surface, two disparate variable domains may seem unsatisfactory or even presumptuous. The above information was a result of analyses that were done after the fact, long after the data were collected. However, it is clear from the data presented in this chapter, and the work of Holinger and Offer (1982) and Holinger et al. (1987) on the direct relationship between cohort size and self-destructive behavior among adolescents, that economic and demographic factors are related to and affect the mental health of a significant number of people. The work of Easterlin was used above in order to illustrate the general relationships between economic and health factors, as well as some theoretical notions concerning these factors.

While we appear to have come up with some interesting facts concerning the relationship between two social worlds—the economic (including the demographic), and the psychological—we are aware of the tenuousness of our findings. As interesting as these kinds of cross-sectional studies are, they are like road signs—one may not be sufficient to get to the desired destination. In other words, more studies like ours are necessary before we can be more certain that the relationships we described above are scientifically valid.

CHAPTER 5

Discussion
Becoming an Adult in the World

*Why, then the world's mine oyster, which
I with sword will open.*

—William Shakespeare, *The Merry Wives
of Windsor*

The "Universal Adolescent" • *The Emergence of a "Global
Village"* • *The Influence of Media* • *Gender, Age, and National
Differences* • *Toward a Common Developmental Psychology of
Adolescents* • *Epilogue*

A major finding of this book is that adolescents from diverse countries and cultures can be understood by psychologically using a structured personality test. Thus studied, they express many common feelings, concerns, and interests.

This assertion seems to clash with the position of many cultural relativists. A generation ago that point of view seemed predominant. The emphasis among anthropologists was on unique cultures. The theoretical position of classical cultural relativists like Benedict (1934) and Mead (1928) was that human populations vary widely in their cultural values, and in their moral and ethical conceptions. To understand a culture other than one's own, they asserted, requires seeing it from an indigenous point of view. Relativists typically hold that cultural differences are so pervasive that there is hardly any basis for cross-cultural comparison. They also take to task psychologists who ethnocentrically presumed the universality of patterns of child rearing, personality development, and sex-role behavior. They tried to show, ultimately, that personality patterns were integral parts of the cultural configurations that gave them meaning (LeVine, 1982).

An example of the cultural relativist viewpoint is seen in the theoretical stance of certain ethnographers and linguists who describe not only differences in customs or artifacts but fundamental differences in world view across cultures. They hold that assumptions about the universe—which differ from one culture to another—are embedded in language, even though speakers of that language might not be fully aware of those assumptions. For example, Dorothy Lee (1950) described a tribe (Wintu Indians) who spoke a language that did not include nouns that referred to specific and discrete entities. Wintu Indians, consequently, did not conceive of themselves or other objects as discrete entities. Instead, they referred to and thought about themselves as adjectives modifying a continuous space or reality. Thus, whereas a Western person might refer to himself as John Smith, a Wintu Indian might refer to himself as the John-Smithish person. According to Lee, this linguistic difference translated into a completely different view of self in society. Instead of viewing themselves as completely separate from others and the world, Wintu Indians appear to have thought of themselves as intimately connected with, though different in a quantitative way from, the rest of the universe. As a result, attitudes toward others and the physical world among Wintu Indians differed sharply from those of their Western counterparts. Extreme cultural relativists hold that persons cannot be understood without a deep immersion in the language, values, and folkways of their culture.

The data in this book stand in opposition to the cultural relativist position. Our data indicate that adolescents in much of the world do not have difficulty understanding one another. The era of impediments to understanding among mutually arcane or alien cultures is largely a matter of the past.

THE "UNIVERSAL ADOLESCENT"

We described adolescents from ten countries. We discussed their psychological self-portraits, focusing on both their differences and their similarities. In this chapter we are going to move beyond the data and speculate on the meaning of these empirical findings.

Similarities among the adolescents whom we studied constitute a portrait of the "universal adolescent." This portrait comprises important aspects of all the selves—psychological, social, sexual, familial, and coping.

Universal adolescents describe themselves this way: (1) Psychologically, they are happy most of the time. They enjoy life. In their view, when others look at them they do not see persons who are poorly developed. They perceive themselves as able to exercise self-control. (2) At a social level, universal adolescents are caring and oriented toward others. They care about how others might be affected by the adolescents' actions. They do not prefer to be alone, and they derive a good feeling from being with others. They feel that there is plenty they can learn from others. (3) Universal adolescents value work and school. They enjoy doing a job well and think about the kind of work that they will do in the future. They would rather work than be supported. They consider school and studying to be important. (3) Universal adolescents express confidence about their sexual selves. Sexually, they do not feel they are far behind. They are not afraid to think or talk about sex. They do not feel they are boring to the opposite sex. (4) Positive feelings toward their families are expressed by universal adolescents. They feel that both parents are basically good, and that they will not be disappointed in or ashamed of their offspring in the future. Mutual esteem is expressed in that they do not carry a grudge against their parents, and they feel that their parents are usually patient and satisfied with them most of the time. Reflecting a positive view of the family, universal adolescents perceive their parents as getting along well with each other most of the time. (5) Coping also represents a positive area for universal adolescents. They feel they can cope with life's vicissitudes. They are able to make decisions, feel talented, and like to put things in order and make sense of them. When faced with a problem, universal adolescents try to find out as much as possible about it in advance in order to cope with it more effectively. If they fail, they try to find out what can be done about that to avoid another failure. They are confident in that they feel certain that they will be able to assume responsibility for themselves in the future.

Recalling the theories cited in Chapter 2, it can be concluded that universal adolescents have mastered many tasks from a Freudian perspective. They are able to cope effectively with sexual and aggressive drives. They have been able to achieve reasonable narcissism, being able to learn from others, for instance, and cope with failure effectively. Regarding a central task of adolescence, effective separation from one's family of origin, these universal adolescents apparently are doing well. They feel positive toward their parents and believe that the parents feel the same way about them. They are not angry at their parents, and they expect to act in ways in the future that will lead the parents to continue to feel good about their offspring. From other perspectives, too, universal adolescents are doing well. They are realistic and oriented toward the future (Kelly, 1955). They are oriented toward others and want to learn from them (Bandura, 1977; Berger and Luckmann, 1966). They react to new social situations with self-control and self-regulation

(Bandura, 1977; Mischel, 1977). Universal adolescents are attuned to cognitive mastery, showing ability to reflect, reason, and think critically on new intellectual levels (Piaget, 1967). Moral values are asserted by universal adolescents, such as affirmation regarding the importance of telling the truth (Kohlberg and Gilligan, 1971). Perhaps, as significant, it is this affinity toward telling the truth that leads us to believe that it is the authentic self of the universal adolescent that we measured (reference from Chapter 2) and not just an adult-pleasing presented self (Goffman, 1959).

Universal adolescents also stand for an affirmation of Chomsky's views regarding the possibility of core aspects of the self across cultures. When the many apparent layers of human diversity are peeled away (like language, race, or religion), we are left with core attitudes and values that motivate and guide many of us. In Chomsky's (1975) terminology, the "surface structure" varies, but the "deep structure" of the self is similar. The definition of self ("that which a person is really and intrinsically"), and the original meaning of psyche ("animating force"), characterizes a core self that transcends differences among adolescents in many nations.

Sources for the "universal adolescent" experience are the biological, cognitive, and developmental aspects of being human. Biological development offers relatively clear characteristics that distinguish childhood from adolescence. Physical changes are universal, though the overlap in timing between the onset of puberty and social recognition of the status of adulthood is socially determined. Cognitive psychology has universal constructs, such as formal operations (Piaget, 1967), that can be used conceptually and empirically to distinguish children's, adolescents', and adults' functioning.

Developmental tasks include developing a clear, coherent view of self and separating from one's family of origin. Adolescents also must learn how to relate to others of a like age and to prepare to form a conjugal family of their own. In addition, they must develop a viable social identity that will synthesize personal characteristics with an acceptable social role (Erikson, 1950; Offer and Offer, 1975).

One universal characteristic of adolescents that is often ignored is the excitement of being an adolescent—an excitement that concerns the movement away from childhood toward increasing skills, forming new relationships, and achieving the important role of socially accepted adult. Bearing witness to this characteristic are rituals marking the transition from childhood to adulthood during early adolescence. These rituals seem pervasive, if not universal. They differ greatly in form but have in common the recognition and celebration of the increased physical and mental power and the elevated status that accompanies the transition from childhood. The areas of agreement we found are notable in this context. In the transition from childhood to adulthood, universal adolescents are able and ready. They stand with their peers but also have a close alliance with their families. They have self-control and feel able to master their environment. They are forward-looking and eager to meet the future.

Indications of a universal adolescent self contrast with the relative dearth of studies in the literature focusing on psychological development from a cross-cultural perspective. There are only a few studies on adolescents in other cultures: Ezeiloi (1982), Franco (1983), Fry (1974), Furnham and Karris (1983), Hille (1981), Olowu (1983), Rodriguez, Behar, Martinez, and Barioud (1982), and Smith, Weigart, and Thomas (1979). Considering the breadth and inherent interest of the subject matter, the relative paucity of studies is remarkable.

While comparative studies of adolescents from diverse cultures have been sporadic in the past, it is our belief that studies like ours will increase considerably in the next decades. They are easier to execute, analyze, and interpret. Psychological instruments, although often tied to their own culture, are becoming less and less parochial.

In the next section we will discuss the factors that, in our opinion, have made it possible for adolescents from diverse cultures to experience their psychological worlds in similar ways, and have made it easier for researchers to describe that commonality.

THE EMERGENCE OF A "GLOBAL VILLAGE"

Twenty years ago McLuhan said that the electronic interdependence caused by the communication revolution has recreated the world in the image of a "global village." McLuhan's thesis is that "the medium, or process, of our time—electric technology—is reshaping and restructuring patterns of social interdependence and every aspect of our personal life. It is forcing us to reconsider and reevaluate practically every thought, every action, and every institution formerly taken for granted." He also said:

> Societies have always been shaped more by the nature of the media by which men communicate than by the content of the communication. . . . The alphabet and print technology fostered and encouraged a fragmenting process, a process of specialism and detachment. Electric technology fosters and encourages unification and involvement. (McLuhan and Fiore, 1967, p. 8)

A new term has come into existence to describe what the world is currently experiencing—the *telemicroelectronic revolution* (TMER).

TMER is an important aspect of the rapid social change that is destined to reach every country on the globe (Lonner, 1985). Television is a significant part of this revolution. Profound changes have indeed occurred in all societies around the world as a result of the proliferation of technological advancements. Nations are no longer isolated in their struggle to face problems of hunger and poverty or injustice. Mass media have made the world into one intercommunicating whole. Not only has one nation's awareness of other nations grown, but also one nation's concern for another. It is McLuhan's view that "youth instinctively understands the present environment—the electric drama. It lives mythically and in depth" (McLuhan and Fiore, 1967, p. 9). It will prove productive and enlightening to reconsider McLuhan's view as we enter the 1990s. Our results, however, indicate that among teenagers, to a meaningful degree, the "global village" exists in the here and now. We can discern a surprising unity of adolescent experience.

Two images govern much contemporary thinking about psychology and social life, according to Sennett (1977). One image is of collective personality, and the other is of collective consciousness. Sennett defines collective personality as the ability of people to interact with each other, to share sensations, to perform common actions, and to share an essential likeness that is understood through reflectively recognizing common characteristics in another person. Collective consciousness involves the ability of people to interact without having to imagine this collective person of whom they all are part.

There may be no better illustration of these two images than the account given by Mead (1978) of her experience in New Guinea. Mountain men, who had washed the pig fat out of their hair, arrived, naked, at a government post, saying, "We have built a school and hospital. Please send us a doctor and a teacher" (p. 121). They were calling for emissaries from the modern world that they had heard about and desired to experience more directly.

A number of social scientists—for example, Erikson (1964), Geertz (1973), G. H. Mead (1934), M. Mead (1978), and Rogers (1980)—have also asserted that the notion of cultural relativity will be soon replaced by a common perspective of interdependence. Their writings elaborate upon the notion of psychic unity. They are implying that humankind will come to realize that it shares personal values, knowledge, ethical standards, and even a common psychosociocultural goal. Although their words and descriptions differ, the psychological meaning of their statements are almost identical. Erikson says, for example: "In our time, for the first time, one human species can be envisaged, with one common technology on one globe. . . . The nature of history is about to change. . . . Joint survival demands that man visualize new ethical alternatives" (Erikson, 1964, pp. 156–157).

THE INFLUENCE OF MEDIA

It is of historical interest to note that as early as 1916 Wundt had outlined a metatheoretical vision of history's four main periods focused around the concept of "folk psychology." Folk psychology, Wundt theorized, was the true "psychology of mankind." Wundt stated that the history of mankind will go through four periods: (1) primitive man; (2) the totemic age; (3) the age of heroes and gods, and, finally; (4) the development to humanity. In each of these periods, culture has to undergo major evolutionary steps, paralleling the psychological advances of mankind. According to Wundt, this final period—the development to humanity—has already begun to take place through the rise of world empires, the development of a world culture, the rise of world religions, and a world history through which the whole of humanity becomes conscious of its unity.

In Wundt's concept of a world culture, we have the basis for the emergence of a universal self—that is, a core self that would have in common elements of human nature, culture, and civilization. This universal self is based on human beings' having come in contact with and assimilated a pattern of meanings that have been dispersed and spread throughout the world. The universal self, then, would have a body of knowledge that is shared by many people across cultures.

Today's teenagers share both a collective personality and a collective consciousness. They watch airplanes in the sky above them, listen to the radio, and watch a rocket launched on TV. They think of these as everyday events. A 14-year-old in Bangladesh may watch the same television program as a 14-year-old in West Germany, Israel, Japan, Turkey, or Taiwan. Media knows no borders; ideas and events are transmitted to all corners of the globe, defining what is new or desirable, and are assimilated by young minds.

The cultural and educational role of television on a global scale is just beginning to be understood. Granzberg (1985) has observed that, bombarded daily by seductive "Hollywood" images of the plentitude of Western ways and the comparative backwardness of non-Western ways, people in developing countries undergo an experience analogous to that encountered by subjects who have a mirror held up before them—they experience heightened awareness of themselves in contrast to these Western images. Western man also has responded to Eastern images, realizing, for instance, that free market individualism contrasts with differing Eastern visions of duty to family, enterprise, and nation.

Television may be functioning "as a type of significant other" on the global level. Newton and Buck (1985) found that television's importance for viewers is not a function of how often television is watched but is a function of what television "tells" viewers about themselves. The image of self that television helps to construct differs for the sexes: gender differences outnumbered cross-cultural differences. Their findings support the notion that the image of ideal others that television helps to construct may be very similar across cultures, though different for males and females.

Contemporary researchers are noticing fewer differences between cultures, owing in part to the vast influence of television and other global communications. Television itself serves as a universal influence on the developing self, displacing certain kinds of more traditional activities. Evidence indicates that watching television displaces participation in community activities, such as sports, dances, and parties, especially for youths (Williams, 1985). This could mean that instead of becoming more like their local cohorts by interacting with them at activities outside of school, teenagers may be assimilating more of what their cohorts in other parts of the world are assimilating. This process of assimilation may be creating something like a global cohort of teenagers around the world that are being influenced by information and images having a common origin. We can now say that though they may not be aware of it as such, or say it to themselves, today's teenagers are experiencing what Wundt had envisioned some seven decades ago as a world culture.

It does appear, then, that we do live in a "global village," as McLuhan proclaimed. The signs are much more evident as we near the final decade of the twentieth century. We are witnessing a process that is becoming more obvious each year. The process we are pointing out is one that will in all likelihood have an even greater impact on the generation of teenagers to follow this one. That is why we feel it most important to emphasize this now, because it is a phenomenon that will only grow in importance; the "global village" we can now get a glimpse of will become even more real in the decades to come.

It may be that the teenagers of the 1980s and beyond, especially those in the developing, non-Western countries, are among the first who really have grown up with a sense of comradery with teenagers from other parts of the world. They are probably more aware that some of what they are experiencing has also been experienced by other teen-agers around the world. The idea of a "global" cohort would not have been possible to consider a decade or two ago. In the 1980s, we were able to collect our data from 5,938 adolescents from ten diverse countries. This "global" cohort of middle-class teenagers represents at least a beginning of a reaching out for a representative sample from these countries.

Recently, the pendulum seems to have swung away from cultural relativism and toward a more universalist position. It would not be surprising if the vanguard of this movement were among teenagers. It is a bit ironic that the world view we find emerging now is in some ways very close to the type held for many generations by the Wintu Indians. The advancement of technology throughout the Western nations has made it possible for us to, in a sense, "catch up with" the traditional wisdom of many folk groups.

We do not wish to appear unaware that there is currently a strong tendency in many areas of the world toward intense nationalism or other forms of chauvinism. Many peoples feel they have not achieved the autonomy or recognition they deserve. Differences on the basis of religion, language, and historical experience become the basis for intense national strivings. Our data, however, lead us to feel it is more important to emphasize the many commonalities we have found. Our data emphasize the universal, not the divisive, and, given the fact that youth are the future of all societies, universality, not divisiveness, may be the wave of the future.

GENDER, AGE, AND NATIONAL DIFFERENCES

Describing the "universal adolescent" does not deny the importance of differences by demographic grouping as well as at the individual level. Our results do point to important gender, age, and national differences among adolescents.

One of our more striking findings is the consistent difference in self-image between adolescent boys and adolescent girls. They were of considerably larger magnitude than were the differences between younger and older adolescents. We cannot, nor do we believe anyone at the present time can, determine the overall influence of biological and sociocultural factors in causing these differences in self-image. The evidence concerning the role that hormones have on the behavior of adolescents is not clearly understood. Although testosterone tends to increase aggressivity and estrogen tends to decrease aggressive behavior, the hormones interact with powerful psychosocial stimuli that are embedded in child-rearing practices and in cultural attitudes toward males and females.

One way of understanding gender differences is to understand them historically, by attending to deeply entrenched cultural, religious, and mythological roots. Evidence indicates that different social roles were performed by males and females in all known societies (Harris, 1974). The hunter and warrior ideal was the one that was typical for males. The hunter and warrior must have good impulse control. He does not give in to his emotions because he must control himself and plan carefully in order to conquer his prey or opponent. He masters his feelings—planning and waiting for the opportune moment to act. In our samples, boys saw themselves as proud of their bodies and morally opportunistic. They more often stated, "I do not care how my actions affect others as long as I gain something." In contrast, boys were less prone than were girls to report adherence to social cooperation. Yet, cooperating, as well as competing with others, is part of being a good hunter or warrior. To be successful, one needs to be able to function in a group as well as be a "lone hunter" or "lone warrior." Cooperating and competing are both abilities that a warrior or hunter had to possess in order to be successful. Many boys seem to adhere more to the competitive than to the cooperative aspects of the traditional male role.

Girls expressed more emotional vulnerability and social commitment than did boys. The image presented by girls conforms to the archetype of the nurturing, domestic preserver of the social fabric. The nurturer and keeper of the hearth can be emotionally expressive and vulnerable because her focus is on consolidating relationships and increasing the level of intimacy within the family. Girls' adherence to more conservative sexual attitudes similarly fits with a primary commitment to the family unit. An important traditional attribute of conjugal families is a commitment to sexuality only within that unit. Sexuality outside the conjugal family tends to destabilize and threaten that unit. From this point of view, girls' commitment to traditional values, such as work and school, can be readily understood.

Less easy to explain is that girls much more often reported feeling ugly and unattractive than did boys. Stereotypically, girls in the traditional, nurturing, and domestic role would very much want to be sexually attractive, since attractiveness would help consolidate the conjugal family unit. If girls were merely presenting a stereotype of femininity, it would be expected that they would be more likely than the boys to report feeling attractive, not unattractive. Their reporting unattractiveness may reflect the insecurity and anxiety associated with the relatively low status and powerlessness of women in many societies throughout the world.

Contrasts by age were expectable in a sense, since they appeared to reflect increasing maturity within the adolescent phase of life. Within the context of positive findings regarding self-image across the teenage years, we found greater self-confidence and greater openness to feedback from others among older as opposed to younger adolescents. These data, we believe, reinforce prior findings (Offer and Offer, 1975) that there is a smooth transition from childhood to adulthood for the vast majority of adolescents. The "turmoil" of the young teenager is the obverse of their hopefulness and enthusiasm. The lack of knowledge about one's capabilities and standing in society is a source of both hope and anxiety. Most adolescents cope with this mixed-feeling state by initiating and assimilating experiences with others so that with the passage of time a solid foundation of reasonable self-evaluation is built. During the transition time, confidence may be somewhat low. With the foundation of positive experiences with others, older adolescents are able to appreciate and draw from others without feeling diminished in contrast. They feel secure about experiences that used to be frightening, such as sexual feelings and aggressive activities. The implication of these data is not that young teenagers are in the throes of tortured self-doubt and frightening lack of control of impulses. Instead, the implication is that the young are uncertain but are gradually finding their way; the older adolescent is more sure and is steadily reaching toward the maturity of adulthood.

Regarding national differences, perhaps most striking was the influence of demographic factors. Very likely reflecting the extreme poverty of their nation, Bengali youths consistently attested to more emotionality, sadness, and loneliness than youths from other countries. Our statistical analysis shows a strong correlation between a nation's gross national product (GNP) and the emotional tone scale, or mood, of that nation's youths. At the same time, the coping ability of teenagers in any country must never be forgotten. Bengali youths scored among the highest of youths in any country studied with respect to superior adjustment. They may be economically poor relative to adolescents in the other countries studied, but, like youth everywhere, their course is forward and their vision is toward an improving future.

Of interest in our results was the relatively strong relationship between one demographic variable—proportion of adolescents in the total population (adolescent density)—and aspects of adolescent self-image. We would like to review in more detail now one theory that is particularly relevant to this finding.

Easterlin (1980) described the special social problems that confront birth cohorts of large size. Utilizing cohort analysis, he and Brenner (1979) suggested using population and economic variables to predict a variety of physical, social, and psychological problems. In a recent conference sponsored by the Institute of Medicine (1985), Easterlin's hypothesis was summarized. The basic hypothesis states that there is a cause–effect relationship between birth cohort size and economic, social, educational, and political trends. Specifically, it correlates movements in birth rates and age-specific rates with particular behavioral phenomena. According to Easterlin, when the size of the birth cohort increases, it produces excessive competition for existing and limited resources in institutions and results in relative deprivation.

Once members of the baby-boom generation reach the labor market, they are likely to meet an unfavorable situation, since a large number of entrants are competing for relatively few opportunities. Having come from a similar situation in the family and schools, these individuals may not have the personal or educational resources needed to compete for limited jobs. As a result, in comparison with smaller cohorts, their relative earnings deteriorate, and their upward mobility is adversely affected. In an effort to improve their economic conditions, members of a larger cohort may exhibit adaptive behaviors such as trying to improve their educational status, delaying marriage, reducing the number of children they have, and having both spouses working. These stresses may also result in antisocial behavior, such as drug and alcohol abuse, and crime.

The birth cohort theory of Easterlin and Brenner was applied by Holinger, Offer, and Ostrov (1987) toward understanding the epidemiology of adolescent suicide. A significant correlation, in the United States, between adolescent suicide rate and the proportion of adolescents in the total population was reported by them. For an older age group (59–65 years old), the opposite relationship was found; for example, an increase in the proportion of older people was associated with a decrease in their suicide rates. Since the proportion of adolescents in the population can be determined years in advance, these findings create the potential for predicting adolescent suicide rates. On the basis of this model, for example, it was predicted that the adolescent suicide rate would level off and decrease throughout the 1980s and into the mid-1990s, at which time another increase should begin (Holinger, Offer, and Zola, 1987). Recent preliminary data of suicide rates have supported this expectation. Thus, the demographic characteristics of adolescents within a specific country is of great importance, with impact not only on economic factors but on mental health factors as well. In our study, Turkey and Bangladesh have the highest proportion of adolescents in the total population. This is probably one of the factors that contributed to the relatively low self-image of adolescents in those countries.

Findings of differences secondary to gender, age, and birth cohort size across various categories of adolescence does not nullify the central finding of our study, which concerns the universality of adolescent experience. Our data most clearly fit in with the "universal" point of view. We were able to find large areas of common experience among teenagers living in widely disparate cultural environments. These findings, we acknowledge, reflect the spirit of our times, a movement away from cultural relativism and toward finding commonalities of human experience. But they probably also reflect an actual increasing homogenization of cultures and, in particular, the experience of adolescence throughout the world.

TOWARD A COMMON DEVELOPMENTAL PSYCHOLOGY OF ADOLESCENTS

The results presented in this book should come as no surprise to anyone familiar with our previous work (Offer, 1969; Offer and Offer, 1975; Offer, Ostrov, and Howard, 1981a). Despite the fact that we have consistently demonstrated that most adolescents grow up mentally healthy and without emotional turmoil, this fact has not been accepted by everyone.

In our previous studies of adults working with adolescents (Offer, Ostrov, and Howard, 1981b; Hartlage, Howard, and Ostrov, 1984), we found that psychiatrists, psychologists, and other professionals working with teenagers describe normal or mentally healthy adolescents as moody and rebellious, and in constant emotional turmoil. They believe normal teenagers' behavior borders on the delinquent, and that they have poor coping abilities. It is striking to note that despite recent studies showing that normal adolescents relate well to family and adults and are free of serious psychopathology (see Offer et al., 1981a), the mental health literature still describes adolescents as impulse-ridden, problematic, without realistic goals, and with poor relationships with their families (see, e.g., Diagnostic and Statistical Manual of Mental Disorders, 1980).

Much of world literature asserts that adolescents cannot be trusted, are often dangerous or suicidal, and are incredibly self-centered. From ancient times to the present, the older generation has been uncomfortable about its young. The reasons are complex. One factor may involve older generations' seeing in youth their own demise and the erosion of their coveted values. Another may involve failure of older persons to understand new trends that adolescents exemplify. In any event, it is the reality, not the myth, of adolescents that we should seek to know. Concern about adolescents has not been matched by sufficient valid, systematic data collection.

A case in point involves adults' perceptions of youths' concern with nuclear war (Lifton, 1985). Although a certain percentage of adolescents are indeed concerned about nuclear issues, they are in the minority—19% of a random group of students from three Chicago high schools (Offer, Ostrov, and Howard, 1986a). The sense one gets is that many adults take the position that adolescents all over the world are deeply concerned, even preoccupied, with the imminent demise of civilization as we know it; if it is not through nuclear war that the world will be destroyed, then it is through thinning of the ozone layer or increases in AIDS. Developmentally, adults may find it easier to face their own death if they believe that death is imminent for everybody, not just themselves. Prophesies of impending doom, judgment day, or major holocausts are almost universal and are found among the beliefs held in many religions (Eliade, 1963). In contemporary times, we have our own prophets of doom who focus on the destruction of Earth through eventualities such as a "nuclear winter." In fact, there is no incontrovertible evidence that a nuclear winter would result from a nuclear war (Marshall, 1987). Despite this lack of scientific certainty, various scholars have taken a strong stand that life on this planet is on the threshold of extinction.

Theoretical notions concerning death have always held a strong attraction for individuals from diverse backgrounds. Psychoanalysts have talked about the death instinct, existential philosophers about the apprehension of each of us regarding our own demise. Adults perceive that the time remaining before death represents a decreasing proportion of their total expectable life-span. The past looms larger and their future becomes proportionally smaller.

Adolescents, in contrast, are just beginning life as fully sentient beings. Their outlook is forward, not backward; they look forward to becoming, not ceasing to be. For most adolescents death is a concept, or an experience, that is relatively foreign. Most of them are not worried about a possible nuclear winter (Offer, Ostrov, and Howard, 1986a). To put the matter another way, mortality is not a typical adolescent issue. On the whole, adolescents do not have the need to project their own apprehensions about mortality to a concern about the destruction of the human race.

Forecasts of doom and destruction have been so appealing to so many peoples over the centuries, at least in part, because adults generalize from the psychology appropriate to their stage in life. By contrast, the hopefulness and enthusiasm of adolescents is appropriate to their stage in life. The contrast between what adolescents feel and what adults believe they must be feeling emphasizes, in our opinion, why it is so important to collect data from adolescents themselves. Our theories concerning the developmental psychology of adolescents have evolved from empirical data. They have allowed us to question some universally accepted theories of adolescent development, such as adolescent turmoil (Offer, 1969; Offer et al., 1981a), and to present new and different notions.

It goes without saying that the empirical approach does not always hold sway. People are invested in their own belief systems and are not easily moved. Many adults hold entrenched beliefs that most adolescents harbor nothing but ill feelings toward adults in general and their parents in particular. Teenagers are felt to be basically "no good" and to symbolize to adults that doomsday is indeed around the corner. Further, they believe that since the young are our future, our future is bleak indeed. The position of the adult appraising youth without a solid empirical foundation is like the person described in this quote: "The pessimist will continue, as in the past, to be convincing in argument, but wrong in fact" (Forbes, 1951).

EPILOGUE

We would like to address the individuals in the adult world who relate directly to teenagers—parents, teachers, counselors, and mental health workers—as well as teenagers themselves, and present what we see as two possible scenarios for the world's teenagers in the next decade and beyond.

We are currently at a crucial transition point in the social-psychological development of adolescents. As seen in this book, middle-class adolescents from diverse cultures have, on the whole, more in common with one another than might have been thought to be the case. The ability to communicate freely and to understand others might lead to a better, more hopeful world in the near future. However, there also exists much hunger, disease, and discontent worldwide. There are also conflicting ideologies. Even in our middle-class sample, about 20% were unhappy and disturbed adolescents. We know that the potential for aggression can erupt at any time. After all, we are only 42 years removed from the end of World War II, when millions of people lost their lives.

The world has always been at a crossroads between cooperative progress on the one hand, and chaos and conflict on the other. The communication revolution has brought people closer together, but it also has the potential of increasing discontent for those who lack material and/or psychosocial goods, for the simple reason that they can now be acutely aware of what they do not have.

Returning to our data, our middle-class population is divided into two groups in dealing with their psychological world. One group is happy most of the time, thinks about the kind of work they will do in the future, and cares about others. The other group is frequently sad, very lonely, empty emotionally, finds no solution to life's endless problems, and may even rather die than go on living.

The disturbed group are the depressed, sometimes "quietly disturbed," adolescents of our study. They tend to be socially alienated, to have difficulty coping, and generally to have a poor self-image. They really have not found their place in the world. A number of factors may currently be causing this in the wide range of national settings we have looked at. Poverty and deprivation are factors, as are cultural upheaval and transformation. Having not one, but many competing value systems can create a great struggle for the adolescent in maintaining a sense of sameness and continuity. This loss of community tradition and family cohesivesness can contribute significantly to the difficult search for identity.

"Quietly disturbed," or depressed, adolescents very likely experience self-doubt, and the prospect of too many decisions and commitments all at once may be too much for them, resulting in confusion and possible psychopathology. Or, if their depression takes the form of scorn or hostility toward the roles offered them, they may behave in a rebellious manner that might lead to unhappiness and self-destructiveness.

A healthy adolescent self-image characterizes at least 73% of the teenagers studied. They would seem to be moving toward adulthood with a healthy integration of previous experiences, self-confidence, a sense of continuity, and optimism regarding career goals. This group has a relatively high degree of endorsement of items that indicate social concern. This healthy, or "universal" adolescent may be well on the way to adjusting to the emerging world view of our time. We might say that today's teenagers may be the first to have begun their reasoning lives with an awareness of the "shared vision," and a "widening fellowship with strong work commitments" that Erikson (1977, p. 148) noted. This trend may overwhelm regressive trends toward conflict and chaos.

A new generation is growing up not only with a knowledge of technological and scientific advancements but with a parallel concern for others as well. It may be that the adolescent of the future will be characterized by an awareness of the interrelatedness of all peoples. In many societies of the past, the village was the world. Today, and tomorrow even more so, many teenagers appear to be recognizing that the world is their community.

Now that we have traveled down the road of exploring the self-image of thousands of adolescents in ten countries throughout the world, our feeling is one of optimism rather than pessimism. When asked, youths willingly share their inner world. They share feelings and thoughts that reflect their vibrancy and eagerness to assume adult roles. Our feeling, after listening to them, is reciprocal to theirs. We are happy that it is they who will inherit the earth.

Commentary

Interest in the self is as old as the science of psychology. William James in 1890 had much to say about it. While interest diminished during psychology's behaviorist period (up to about 1950), it has reemerged with spectacular intensity. This volume is in a solid tradition.

Cooley defined the self as all the sentences that people use that contain the words *I, me, mine,* or *myself.* This is a very large universe of cognitions. People sample this universe differently from moment to moment, depending on the situation: who the other in the situation is, what the other just did, and who they are. In this volume the authors tell us how the "who they are" affects the self. The subjects are asked to rate how self-relevant various self-related cognitions are. Almost 6,000 subjects from ten countries provided ratings to about 100 such cognitions. Thus, a segment of the self was measured. This segment has five aspects: (1) the psychological, such as emotions and feelings about the self; (2) the social, such as the person's sociability; (3) the sexual; (4) the familial; and (5) the coping self. The data were treated in a sophisticated manner by eliminating items that did not behave properly in all cultures and by looking for patterns of consistent responses across all cultures.

The search for universal aspects of the self was carried out very well. Taking advantage of the relatively short time required from each person, the authors collected data from large samples, with standard stimuli, so the responses could be compared.

The authors show a sophisticated understanding of the limitations of their approach. They know that the teenager can provide responses only to questions specifically posed. There is no opportunity to inquire about aspects of the subject's world that are specific to particular cultures. The authors interpret results only when there is consistency across samples.

At times, however, the authors use language that is not justified. For example, the talk about a "universal adolescent," in the last chapter, is not entirely accurate because they sampled teenagers who were literate, urban, middle class, and exposed to the mass media. That still is a minority of mankind. The most dramatic cross-cultural differences that I know of have been obtained when comparing literate and nonlite-rate samples. Unfortunately, much of the population in less developed countries is still illiterate. The image of cultural conversion that the authors present may be an illusion due to their particular sampling. Yes, middle-class adolescents may think alike, but these teenagers may be diverging progressively from teenagers in their cultures who are less affluent. Without representative samples we cannot say much about a "universal adolescent." Thus, I would have preferred the wording "the adolescents in our samples."

I am also not too happy with the extent to which the authors relied on percentages. Percentages are much more susceptible to variations due to sampling than are means. A representative sample may still give the same means as their sample of convenience, while the percent who agree with an item may shift. Also, one must be much more careful with data from single items than with data from scales. I find the dis-cussion on depression, that uses several items, more convincing than some of the discussions of single items.

On a more constructive note, I find many of the data fascinating. They can be used by future investigators to test their own hypotheses. For example, people interested in the dimensions of cultural variation proposed by Hofstede, such as individualism and power distance, may be able to get insights by examining the data in this book. Hypotheses about the way rapid social change may confuse teenagers seem sup-ported by the data. Specially important, I think, is the finding that the higher the proportion of adolescents in a country's population, the less positive the affect reported by its teenagers.

In summary, this is an important book. While the wording of the last chapter may be overgeneral, and the claims that the authors make may not be fully justified, it provides extremely interesting data and insights, and a useful understanding of the world of many teenagers in ten countries.

Harry C. Triandis
University of Illinois
Champaign, Illinois

Appendixes

The Offer Self-Image Questionnaire (OSIQ): International Version

On the following pages are the ten scales that constitute the International OSIQ. For example, the next page shows the Impulse Control scale and its constituent items. (Item numbers are those used in the OSIQ.) Subsequent pages present the Impulse Control items in the original English or as back-translated into English. Percent endorsements for younger (ages 13–15) males (YM), older (ages 16–19) males (OM), younger females (YF), and older females (OF) for each country are shown for each item. It should be noted that responses to each item are on a scale from 1 to 6. Responses of 1 (describes me very well), 2 (describes me well), or 3 (describes me fairly well) constitute an endorsement of the item. In these tables percentages have been rounded to the nearest whole number. Subsequent pages present the remaining scales, their constituent items, and corresponding percent endorsements.

Psychological Self (PS-1)
SCALE: IMPULSE CONTROL

---

8. I "lose my head" easily. (−)

17. At times I have fits of crying and/or laughing that I seem unable to control. (−)

34. I can take criticism without resentment.

59. Even under pressure I manage to remain calm.

69. I keep an even temper most of the time.

81. I fear something constantly. (−)

123. Usually I control myself.

Note. When items are added to form scale scores, items followed by (−) are reversed so that a response of "1" becomes a "6," a "2" becomes a "5," and so forth. No item is reversed for the percentage endorsement presentation.

ITEM 8

Country	Translation	YM	OM	YF	OF
United States	I lose my head easily.	38	24	31	25
Australia	I lose my head easily.	39	40	40	34
Germany	I lose my head easily.	14	15	19	20
Italy	I lose my cool easily.	42	29	51	40
Israel	I am easily at a loss.	27	23	34	31
Hungary	I lose my head easily.	17	25	16	28
Turkey	I become upset (nervous) easily.	23	22	51	66
Japan	I very often cannot stay still.	—	59	—	57
Taiwan	I lose my temper easily.	44	31	64	41
Bangladesh	I lose my patience easily.	32	32	53	50

ITEM 17

Country	Translation	YM	OM	YF	OF
United States	At times I have fits of crying and/laughing that I seem unable to control.	33	24	51	45
Australia	At times I have fits of crying and/or laughing that I seem unable to control.	45	25	57	48
Germany	Sometimes I have crying or laughing jags that I really can't control.	21	23	34	34
Italy	At times I burst into tears and/laughter that I think I can't control.	37	20	50	45
Israel	At times I have spells of laughter or crying that I have difficulty controlling.	22	21	43	38
Hungary	Occasionally I have an urge to laugh or to cry which I almost cannot control.	26	23	37	46
Turkey	Sometimes I have uncontrollable crying and/laughing fits (crises).	30	26	48	50
Japan	Frequently I become extremely and uncontrollably happy or sad.	—	20	—	46
Taiwan	It seems like I cannot stop whenever I cry or laugh very hard.	29	20	44	31
Bangladesh	At times I feel like laughing or crying so hard that I cannot stop it at all.	58	63	70	69

ITEM 34

Country	Translation	YM	OM	YF	OF
United States	I can take criticism without resentment.	59	73	63	70
Australia	I can take criticism without resentment.	42	57	47	64
Germany	I can accept criticism without feeling insulted (hurt).	68	68	63	76
Italy	I accept critique without discernment.	46	47	43	51
Israel	I can accept criticism without bearing a grudge.	62	72	69	74
Hungary	I can accept criticism without feeling offended.	65	68	71	62
Turkey	I can accept criticism without getting offended (hurt).	68	79	70	76
Japan	I can take criticism without negative feeling.	—	48	—	53
Taiwan	I can take criticism without negative feeling.	67	58	47	58
Bangladesh	I am able to accept criticism easily.	67	69	58	64

ITEM 59

Country	Translation	YM	OM	YF	OF
United States	Even under pressure I manage to remain calm.	79	85	69	72
Australia	Even under pressure I manage to remain calm.	69	83	58	59
Germany	Even under pressure I succeed in remaining calm.	72	60	46	43
Italy	Under pressure I remain calm (I try to).	69	77	64	61
Israel	I succeed in remaining calm even under pressure.	72	75	54	45
Hungary	Sometimes I can keep calm in difficult situations.	83	81	68	69
Turkey	I can be calm even under pressure (stress).	61	74	53	47
Japan	Even under stress I can remain calm.	—	49	—	51
Taiwan	I can still keep calm under pressure.	56	63	67	64
Bangladesh	I am cool under pressure.	64	68	62	75

ITEM 69

Country	Translation	YM	OM	YF	OF
United States	I keep an even temper most of the time.	85	88	81	80
Australia	I keep an even temper most of the time.	70	78	67	72
Germany	Most of the time I am even-tempered.	91	81	80	76
Italy	I am almost always in bad humor.	73	73	65	46
Israel	Most of the time I don't lose control.	85	85	85	74
Hungary	I am mostly well balanced.	84	77	81	68
Turkey	Most of the time I have a calm character.	76	80	76	74
Japan	Usually I am calm and patient.	—	65	—	73
Taiwan	Most of the time, I am easy to get along.	95	92	84	87
Bangladesh	I am able to control my temper most of the time.	71	77	66	73

ITEM 81

Country	Translation	YM	OM	YF	OF
United States	I fear something constantly.	24	16	30	20
Australia	I fear something constantly.	35	40	37	35
Germany	I am constantly afraid of something.	9	7	13	14
Italy	I am always afraid of something.	43	32	50	42
Israel	I am always afraid of something.	27	19	31	32
Hungary	I am always afraid of something.	13	16	19	22
Turkey	I am always afraid of something.	2	19	38	36
Japan	I am always afraid of something.	—	40	—	30
Taiwan	I am always afraid of something.	49	51	62	69
Bangladesh	There is an undefinable fear in my mind at all times.	39	41	40	46

ITEM 123

Country	Translation	YM	OM	YF	OF
United States	Usually I control myself.	90	93	91	93
Australia	Usually I control myself.	83	88	80	87
Germany	I usually control myself.	72	82	62	58
Italy	Usually I control myself.	79	81	76	77
Israel	Generally I am in control.	89	84	92	87
Hungary	Usually I can control myself.	87	80	87	78
Turkey	Generally I can control myself.	82	91	84	91
Japan	Usually I can suppress my feelings.	—	83	—	80
Taiwan	I often control my emotion.	70	75	58	63
Bangladesh	Usually I can control my emtions.	79	83	77	85

12. I feel tense most of the time. (−)

23. I feel inferior to most people I know. (−)

32. Most of the time I am happy.

38. My feelings are easily hurt. (−)

54. I am so very anxious. (−)

66. I feel so very lonely. (−)

68. I enjoy life.

100. Even when I am sad I can enjoy a good joke.

130. I frequently feel sad. (−)

ITEM 12

Country	Translation	YM	OM	YF	OF
United States	I feel tense most of the time.	26	28	23	25
Australia	I feel tense most of the time.	24	32	23	26
Germany	I feel pressured most of the time.	23	39	19	40
Italy	I feel I am always tense.	29	27	35	38
Israel	I am tense most of the time.	20	23	26	28
Hungary	I usually feel tense.	16	29	18	29
Turkey	Most of the time I feel tense.	49	46	52	51
Japan	I always feel tense.	—	28	—	30
Taiwan	I often feel tense.	55	37	47	57
Bangladesh	At most times I feel a mental pressure.	52	64	62	74

ITEM 23

Country	Translation	YM	OM	YF	OF
United States	I feel inferior to most people I know.	24	12	18	15
Australia	I feel inferior to most people I know.	30	22	37	18
Germany	I feel inferior to most of the people I know.	12	7	11	1
Italy	I feel inferior to the majority of people I meet.	15	7	23	19
Israel	I feel inferior to most people I know.	16	16	15	7
Hungary	Compared to most of my acquaintances, I have feelings of inferiority.	8	13	8	11
Turkey	I feel inferior to many of the people I know.	20	13	25	21
Japan	I feel that I am lower than my peers.	—	45	—	48
Taiwan	In front of people I know, I often feel inferior.	31	22	20	25
Bangladesh	I feel I am inferior to many people I know.	34	31	32	33

ITEM 32

Country	Translation	YM	OM	YF	OF
United States	Most of the time I am happy.	84	93	85	90
Australia	Most of the time I am happy.	82	80	85	80
Germany	Usually I am happy.	82	74	75	73
Italy	I am almost always happy.	77	65	76	64
Israel	I am happy most of the time.	88	83	83	70
Hungary	I am usually happy.	84	72	89	73
Turkey	Most of the time I am happy.	83	87	80	88
Japan	I am almost always happy.	—	79	—	86
Taiwan	I am happy most of the time.	87	71	82	73
Bangladesh	I am cheerful most of the time.	78	77	81	80

ITEM 38

Country	Translation	YM	OM	YF	OF
United States	My feelings are easily hurt.	33	42	55	56
Australia	My feelings are easily hurt.	46	42	59	61
Germany	My feelings are easily hurt.	22	41	47	54
Italy	My feelings are easily wounded.	47	52	60	59
Israel	My feelings get hurt easily.	45	55	77	74
Hungary	I am easily offended.	23	19	28	38
Turkey	My feelings are easily hurt.	53	55	66	86
Japan	My feelings can get hurt easily	—	64	—	80
Taiwan	My feelings are easily hurt.	29	38	44	63
Bangladesh	I am easily hurt.	60	59	78	80

ITEM 54

Country	Translation	YM	OM	YF	OF
United States	I am so very anxious.	47	53	50	48
Australia	I am so very anxious.	56	53	52	48
Germany	I am very anxious.	6	7	14	11
Italy	I am very anxious.	53	42	58	55
Israel	I am anxious.	9	9	15	17
Hungary	I am very anxious.	17	23	22	25
Turkey	I worry a lot.	38	34	35	46
Japan	I worry very much about almost everything.	—	77	—	69
Taiwan	I am very very anxious.	27	20	24	30
Bangladesh	I am very anxious.	42	40	49	55

ITEM 66

Country	Translation	YM	OM	YF	OF
United States	I feel so very lonely.	14	12	29	19
Australia	I feel so very lonely.	19	23	21	25
Germany	I feel very lonely.	8	11	12	12
Italy	I feel very lonely.	16	14	26	25
Israel	I feel very lonely.	12	18	19	19
Hungary	I feel very lonely.	10	19	10	16
Turkey	I feel very lonely.	31	29	30	35
Japan	I am very lonely.	—	38	—	40
Taiwan	I feel that I am so lonely.	28	37	22	44
Bangladesh	I feel very lonely.	41	32	45	52

ITEM 68

Country	Translation	YM	OM	YF	OF
United States	I enjoy life.	89	97	90	93
Australia	I enjoy life.	88	81	84	78
Germany	I enjoy life.	90	84	83	83
Italy	I love to live.	93	93	88	89
Israel	I enjoy life.	92	88	88	83
Hungary	I enjoy life.	87	79	86	76
Turkey	I enjoy life.	84	92	80	86
Japan	I enjoy my life.	—	67	—	70
Taiwan	I enjoy my life.	71	73	69	70
Bangladesh	I enjoy life.	70	66	78	60

Iтем 100

Country	Translation	YM	OM	YF	OF
United States	Even when I am sad I can enjoy a good joke.	85	85	80	87
Australia	Even when I am sad I can enjoy a good joke.	82	81	73	78
Germany	Even when I am sad I can enjoy a good joke.	73	66	61	60
Italy	Even if I am sad I am entertained by funny stories.	72	66	70	68
Israel	Even when I am sad I can enjoy a good joke.	82	81	76	78
Hungary	I enjoy a good joke even when I am in a bad mood.	79	74	77	68
Turkey	Even if I am sad I enjoy a good joke.	78	82	90	89
Japan	Even when I am sad a good funny joke lifts my spirits.	—	51	—	52
Taiwan	Even when I am sad, I can still enjoy a good joke.	65	58	48	63
Bangladesh	Even if I am sad I enjoy funny jokes.	66	70	56	53

ITEM 130

Country	Translation	YM	OM	YF	OF
United States	I frequently feel sad.	18	20	28	27
Australia	I frequently feel sad.	19	23	32	33
Germany	I feel unhappy a lot.	9	13	24	21
Italy	I am frequently sad.	20	21	35	22
Israel	I am frequently sad.	24	17	31	37
Hungary	I feel sad often.	13	27	21	34
Turkey	I feel sad very often.	35	29	29	40
Japan	I am often sad.	—	54	—	57
Taiwan	I often feel sad.	17	27	24	33
Bangladesh	I am frequently weighed down with sadness.	30	28	40	49

Psychological Self (PS-3)
SCALE: BODY AND SELF-IMAGE

---

27. In the past year I have been very worried about my health. (−)

42. The picture I have of myself in the future satisfies me. (−)

57. I am proud of my body.

72. I seem to be forced to imitate the people I like. (−)

82. Very often I think that I am not at all the person I would like to be. (−)

90. I frequently feel ugly and unattractive. (−)

94. When others look at me they must think that I am poorly developed. (−)

99. I feel strong and healthy.

ITEM 27

Country	Translation	YM	OM	YF	OF
United States	In the past year I have been very worried about my health.	29	23	35	36
Australia	In the past year I have been very worried about my health.	28	27	31	28
Germany	In this past year I worried a lot about my health.	22	17	9	25
Italy	The past years I have been much preoccupied about my health.	35	26	28	25
Israel	In the past year I have been very concerned about my health.	22	16	14	22
Hungary	This past year, I was very worried about my health.	15	17	11	17
Turkey	My health worried me a lot last summer.	27	21	19	26
Japan	Within the past year, I have become more worried about my health.	—	47	—	48
Taiwan	In the past few years, I have been very worried about my health.	49	34	36	30
Bangladesh	I have been anxious about my health for a long time.	59	68	46	52

ITEM 42

Country	Translation	YM	OM	YF	OF
United States	The picture I have of myself in the future satisfies me.	91	79	92	88
Australia	The picture I have of myself in the future satisfies me.	73	76	67	61
Germany	My picture of my future satisfies me.	68	65	61	49
Italy	My future self-image is satisfying.	83	75	78	69
Israel	My image of myself in the future satisfies me.	88	76	72	70
Hungary	The picture I have of myself satisfies me.	65	63	59	47
Turkey	My future image gives me satisfaction (fulfillment).	57	61	48	47
Japan	I will probably be satisfied with my future.	—	35	—	50
Taiwan	I have images of my future, I am satisfied with the images.	65	75	60	73
Bangladesh	Imagining about the future satisfies me.	87	90	85	88

ITEM 57

Country	Translation	YM	OM	YF	OF
United States	I am proud of my body.	81	81	68	72
Australia	I am proud of my body.	75	73	39	38
Germany	I am proud of my body.	73	74	62	61
Italy	I am very proud of my body.	80	75	58	58
Israel	I am proud of my body.	82	75	71	62
Hungary	I am proud of my looks.	42	43	41	36
Turkey	I am proud of my body.	64	79	49	55
Japan	I have confidence in my own body.	—	41	—	23
Taiwan	I am quite satisfied/happy with my body.	65	66	60	56
Bangladesh	I am proud of my physical development.	68	55	59	52

ITEM 72

Country	Translation	YM	OM	YF	OF
United States	I seem to be forced to imitate the people I like.	33	26	28	19
Australia	I seem to be forced to imitate the people I like.	36	35	21	22
Germany	Apparently I have a compulsion to imitate people I like.	13	14	10	9
Italy	I feel like I am forced to imitate people I like.	31	22	27	15
Israel	I feel like I need to imitate the people that I like.	35	34	20	21
Hungary	I feel I should imitate people I love.	44	30	41	32
Turkey	I feel as if I am forced to imitate people that I love.	25	29	16	27
Japan	I seem to be forced to imitate the people I like.	—	12	—	16
Taiwan	I cannot help imitating people I like.	42	63	62	68
Bangladesh	Those that I like, I seem bound to imitate.	61	65	70	58

Iᴛᴇᴍ 82

Country	Translation	YM	OM	YF	OF
United States	Very often I think that I am not at all the person I would like to be.	39	40	37	40
Australia	Very often I think that I am not at all the person I would like to be.	50	52	55	56
Germany	I often think I am not at all the person I want to be.	31	15	41	23
Italy	Frequently I believe I am not the person I would like to be.	35	27	50	41
Israel	Often I think that I am not the person I would like to be.	23	24	30	35
Hungary	Very often I think that I am not at all what I would like to be.	34	46	43	54
Turkey	Most of the time I think I am not the person I want to be.	34	40	46	45
Japan	I believe I am nowhere near the person I want to be.	—	60	—	61
Taiwan	I often think I am not the one I expect to be.	46	47	52	56
Bangladesh	I often think that I am not what I wanted to be.	38	51	56	70

ITEM 90

Country	Translation	YM	OM	YF	OF
United States	I frequently feel ugly and unattractive.	21	17	40	30
Australia	I frequently feel ugly and unattractive.	28	25	50	40
Germany	I often feel ugly and unattractive.	12	9	30	22
Italy	Often I feel ugly and unattractive.	25	23	48	40
Israel	Often I feel ugly and unattractive.	28	22	28	28
Hungary	I often feel I am ugly and unattractive.	25	26	34	34
Turkey	Very often I feel that I am ugly and unattractive.	28	22	34	33
Japan	I feel that I am not attractive because of my looks.	—	51	—	61
Taiwan	I often feel I am ugly and unattractive.	27	26	31	27
Bangladesh	I often think that I am ugly and unattractive.	37	33	30	49

ITEM 94

Country	Translation	YM	OM	YF	OF
United States	When others look at me they must think that I am poorly developed.	16	11	14	8
Australia	When others look at me they must think that I am poorly developed.	15	13	19	16
Germany	When other people look at me they must feel that I am not very developed.	5	5	4	3
Italy	When other people look at me they certainly think I am underdeveloped.	8	5	13	4
Israel	When other people look at me they probably think that I am underdeveloped.	17	12	21	9
Hungary	I am not very mature in the opinion of others.	14	12	10	8
Turkey	When other people look at me they must think that I am not well developed.	34	21	16	12
Japan	Others think I am poorly developed physically.	—	27	—	26
Taiwan	When others see me, they must think that I am poorly developed.	30	18	16	14
Bangladesh	When others see me they must think that my physical form is not good.	28	33	29	29

ITEM 99

Country	Translation	YM	OM	YF	OF
United States	I feel strong and healthy.	85	94	87	88
Australia	I feel strong and healthy.	81	80	67	67
Germany	I feel strong and healthy.	89	84	72	76
Italy	I feel strong and healthy.	83	81	78	71
Israel	I feel strong and healthy.	84	87	87	85
Hungary	I feel strong and healthy.	77	83	83	75
Turkey	I feel strong and healthy.	85	93	83	85
Japan	I feel I am strong and healthy.	—	78	—	82
Taiwan	I feel strong and healthy.	51	63	47	58
Bangladesh	I consider myself healthy and strong.	54	41	47	50

Social Self (SS-1)
SCALE: SOCIAL RELATIONSHIPS

---

13.   I usually feel out of place at picnics and parties. (−)

52.   I think that other people just do not like me. (−)

62.   I find it extremely hard to make friends. (−)

65.   I do not mind being corrected, since I can learn from it.

75.   I prefer being alone (than with other kids my age). (−)

86.   If others disapprove of me I get terribly upset. (−)

88.   Being together with other people gives me a good feeling.

113.   I do not have a particularly difficult time in making friends.

124.   I enjoy most parties I go to.

ITEM 13

Country	Translation	YM	OM	YF	OF
United States	I usually feel out of place at picnics and parties.	27	23	17	23
Australia	I usually feel out of place at picnics and parties.	22	23	19	20
Germany	Most of the time I feel out of place at parties.	12	16	13	11
Italy	Usually at parties I feel that I am out of place.	26	22	32	24
Israel	In general I am not comfortable at parties and picnics.	28	24	25	27
Hungary	Generally, I feel like an outsider in groups and meetings.	15	25	13	18
Turkey	In general, I feel like an outsider at picnics and parties.	45	39	30	35
Japan	I am not comfortable at parties, picnics, and other gatherings.	—	32	—	20
Taiwan	At picnics and parties, I often feel I am not physically there.	36	40	38	43
Bangladesh	At picnics or dinners I am not able to feel comfortable.	34	35	29	33

ITEM 52

Country	Translation	YM	OM	YF	OF
United States	I think that other people just do not like me.	22	13	17	16
Australia	I think that other people just do not like me.	27	24	30	20
Germany	I think that other people do not like me.	27	27	25	9
Italy	I believe I am not liked.	21	16	35	20
Israel	I think that others simply don't like me.	22	14	16	11
Hungary	I believe people don't like me.	12	15	9	17
Turkey	I think that other people don't love me.	47	37	39	47
Japan	Sometimes I feel that other people don't like me.	—	31	—	38
Taiwan	I think other people don't like me.	35	20	29	24
Bangladesh	I think that other people disapprove of me somehow.	28	31	32	17

Iᴛᴇᴍ 62

Country	Translation	YM	OM	YF	OF
United States	I find it extremely hard to make friends.	16	9	8	11
Australia	I find it extremely hard to make friends.	21	14	15	15
Germany	I have great trouble finding friends.	8	10	13	11
Italy	It is difficult for me to make friends.	21	20	26	22
Israel	I find it very hard to be friendly with others.	26	22	12	15
Hungary	I find it extremely difficult to develop friendships.	16	21	8	20
Turkey	I find it very difficult to have friendships.	27	23	30	18
Japan	It is difficult for me to make friends.	—	29	—	25
Taiwan	I have often found that making friends is a difficult task.	20	22	20	25
Bangladesh	Making friends is truly difficult for me.	33	32	32	25

ITEM 65

Country	Translation	YM	OM	YF	OF
United States	I do not mind being corrected, since I can learn from it.	82	85	79	84
Australia	I do not mind being corrected, since I can learn from it.	84	89	81	83
Germany	I do not mind being criticized, because I can learn from it.	77	84	74	80
Italy	It doesn't bother me to stand corrected because I can derive some experience from it.	74	67	69	65
Israel	I don't mind when people make comments, because I can learn from them.	71	73	69	74
Hungary	I do not mind being corrected, because I can learn from it.	84	79	86	79
Turkey	I do not mind being corrected, because I can learn something from it.	47	72	56	68
Japan	I do not mind being corrected, since I can learn from it.	—	52	—	61
Taiwan	I do not mind being corrected, because I can learn from it.	95	87	84	86
Bangladesh	I am not upset if someone corrects my mistakes, for I can learn from them.	90	97	99	98

ITEM 75

Country	Translation	YM	OM	YF	OF
United States	I prefer being alone (than with other kids my age).	29	13	23	24
Australia	I prefer being alone (than with other kids my age).	21	20	13	11
Germany	I would rather be alone than with people my age.	9	9	10	10
Italy	I prefer to be alone than to live with kids my age.	11	5	8	6
Israel	I prefer being alone to being with peers.	21	20	14	12
Hungary	I prefer being alone than being with peers.	13	15	12	16
Turkey	I prefer being alone than being together with my peers.	15	7	11	9
Japan	I would rather be alone than with my peers.	—	22	—	20
Taiwan	I would rather be alone than with people my age.	13	19	13	16
Bangladesh	I prefer to be alone rather than with boys and girls my own age.	20	24	27	32

ITEM 86

Country	Translation	YM	OM	YF	OF
United States	If others disapprove of me I get terribly upset.	31	37	44	42
Australia	If others disapprove of me I get terribly upset.	36	39	47	48
Germany	When others put me down I get terribly upset.	32	42	31	28
Italy	If other people disapprove I get awfully mad.	32	23	34	23
Israel	When others criticize me I get very nervous.	26	14	29	14
Hungary	When someone disagrees with me I get very mad.	13	16	14	17
Turkey	If other people don't agree with (approve of) me, I become upset.	40	39	52	39
Japan	If others disapprove of me I get confused.	—	62	—	74
Taiwan	I feel miserable if someone disagrees with me.	36	45	44	44
Bangladesh	I am very hurt/heartbroken if others do not agree with me.	57	58	60	71

ITEM 88

Country	Translation	YM	OM	YF	OF
United States	Being together with other people gives me a good feeling.	95	98	95	93
Australia	Being together with other people gives me a good feeling.	91	92	92	95
Germany	Being together with others gives me good feelings.	95	89	95	95
Italy	To be with people makes me feel good.	86	83	90	88
Israel	I feel good when I am with others.	85	86	90	89
Hungary	I like to be with other people.	92	91	94	92
Turkey	Being with other people gives me good feelings.	82	95	92	94
Japan	I feel good when I am with my friends.	—	76	—	80
Taiwan	It gives me a good feeling to be with others.	82	80	71	70
Bangladesh	I like mixing with people very much.	90	78	82	85

ITEM 113

Country	Translation	YM	OM	YF	OF
United States	I do not have a particularly difficult time in making friends.	74	89	84	83
Australia	I do not have a particularly difficult time in making friends.	81	79	63	73
Germany	At my age I don't find it hard to make friends.	68	68	60	68
Italy	I do not have any particular difficulties in establishing friendships.	66	63	63	67
Israel	I don't have special difficulties making friends.	81	74	87	80
Hungary	I don't have special difficulties in making friends.	73	69	75	66
Turkey	Especially when making friends, I do not encounter any difficulties (I make friends easily).	74	82	74	87
Japan	I don't think it is difficult to make new friends.	—	67	—	73
Taiwan	In making friends, I have no particular difficulties.	73	66	69	63
Bangladesh	It is not particularly difficult for me to make new friends.	63	69	76	70

ITEM 124

Country	Translation	YM	OM	YF	OF
United States	I enjoy most parties I go to.	84	89	89	86
Australia	I enjoy most parties I go to.	90	84	92	84
Germany	Most of the parties I go to I enjoy.	85	74	88	85
Italy	Usually I am happy at any party I attend.	75	64	74	62
Israel	Generally I enjoy parties.	76	74	86	76
Hungary	I mostly enjoy getting together with friends.	94	89	96	90
Turkey	I enjoy most of the parties I go to.	68	66	83	84
Japan	I can enjoy myself at a party.	—	75	—	89
Taiwan	I enjoyed most of the parties I went to.	50	55	53	47
Bangladesh	I enjoy most of the parties and (social) events that I attend.	80	87	84	89

Social Self (SS-2)
SCALE: VOCATIONAL AND EDUCATIONAL GOALS

---

37. I am sure that I will be proud about my future profession.

46. I would rather sit around and loaf than work. (−)

58. At times I think about what kind of work I will do in the future.

63. I would rather be supported for the rest of my life than work. (−)

70. A job well done gives me pleasure.

79. I feel that there is plenty that I can learn from others. (−)

115. School and studying mean very little to me. (−)

Iᴛᴇᴍ 37

Country	Translation	YM	OM	YF	OF
United States	I am sure that I will be proud about my future profession.	88	89	92	91
Australia	I am sure that I will be proud about my future profession.	89	85	78	79
Germany	I am certain that I will be proud of my future profession.	85	82	74	69
Italy	I am sure I will be proud of my future profession.	81	73	80	69
Israel	I am sure that my future profession will make me proud.	92	84	90	83
Hungary	I am confident that I will be proud of my future vocation.	70	66	69	65
Turkey	I feel that I will be proud of my profession in the future.	90	88	90	89
Japan	I will probably be proud of my job.	—	70	—	74
Taiwan	I truly believe that I will be proud of my job in the future.	64	73	62	66
Bangladesh	I am sure that my profession in the future will be one to be proud of.	82	78	84	67

ITEM 46

Country	Translation	YM	OM	YF	OF
United States	I would rather sit around and loaf than work.	32	24	23	18
Australia	I would rather sit around and loaf than work.	27	23	12	12
Germany	I would rather sit around and loaf than work.	26	24	23	19
Italy	Rather than work I would rather sit and do nothing.	15	15	13	11
Israel	I would prefer sitting and doing nothing to working.	34	32	27	19
Hungary	I would rather sit or goof off than work.	29	45	16	25
Turkey	Rather than working, I prefer to "goof" around and pass the time.	23	20	19	17
Japan	I would rather sit and do nothing than work or study.	—	60	—	46
Taiwan	I would rather loaf and sit around than study hard.	26	23	22	24
Bangladesh	I prefer to spend time sitting around lazily rather than working.	12	21	19	22

ITEM 58

Country	Translation	YM	OM	YF	OF
United States	At times I think about what kind of work I will do in the future.	89	97	95	95
Australia	At times I think about what kind of work I will do in the future.	91	92	89	93
Germany	Sometimes I think about the work I will do in the future.	86	89	94	93
Italy	Frequently I think about the type of work I will do in the future.	85	86	85	93
Israel	Sometimes I wonder what kind of work I will do in the future.	83	83	85	87
Hungary	Sometimes I think about the work I will be doing in the future.	84	84	88	91
Turkey	Sometimes I think about the work I will be doing in the future.	84	89	93	92
Japan	Sometimes I wonder what kind of job I will have.	—	90	—	92
Taiwan	Sometimes I wonder what I will do in the future.	86	91	91	95
Bangladesh	I sometimes think about the kind of work I will do in the future.	95	96	93	89

ITEM 63

Country	Translation	YM	OM	YF	OF
United States	I would rather be supported for the rest of my life than work.	24	12	14	13
Australia	I would rather be supported for the rest of my life than work.	30	18	5	9
Germany	I would rather be supported the rest of my life than work.	6	7	4	3
Italy	I would prefer being supported for the rest of my life instead of working.	9	13	5	5
Israel	I would rather be supported than work all my life.	11	11	9	3
Hungary	I would like to be kept for the rest of my life rather than having to work for a living.	9	15	6	5
Turkey	I would like to live the rest of my life by being supported rather than working.	30	10	8	9
Japan	Rather than work I would like to have someone support me for the rest of my life.	—	12	—	11
Taiwan	I would rather be supported by others for my whole life than to work.	6	7	2	4
Bangladesh	Instead of working myself, the rest of my life I wish to depend of others.	19	9	8	5

ITEM 70

Country	Translation	YM	OM	YF	OF
United States	A job well done gives me pleasure.	94	99	96	100
Australia	A job well done gives me pleasure.	94	98	92	97
Germany	A piece of work well done gives me pleasure.	92	94	93	96
Italy	Work well done is satisfying.	94	98	94	98
Israel	I enjoy completing a task successfully.	98	97	97	99
Hungary	A well-done job makes me glad.	94	93	98	96
Turkey	I enjoy something that is well done.	91	98	96	99
Japan	I am happy when school or work goes well.	—	97	—	100
Taiwan	I feel happy in accomplishing things.	96	95	96	98
Bangladesh	I think neat work.	94	89	98	99

ITEM 79

Country	Translation	YM	OM	YF	OF
United States	I feel that there is plenty that I can learn from others.	88	96	94	98
Australia	I feel that there is plenty that I can learn from others.	83	92	82	90
Germany	I believe I can learn a lot from others.	82	86	83	85
Italy	I believe there are a lot of things I can learn from other people.	87	92	91	92
Israel	I feel that I will be able to learn from others.	76	87	74	83
Hungary	I feel that I can learn a lot from others.	85	88	92	87
Turkey	I feel that I have a lot to learn from other people.	86	90	85	93
Japan	I feel I can learn quite a bit from my friends.	—	94	—	96
Taiwan	I feel I can learn a lot from others.	91	91	96	97
Bangladesh	I think that I can learn much from the actions of others.	88	89	93	90

ITEM 115

Country	Translation	YM	OM	YF	OF
United States	School and studying mean very little to me.	16	12	15	7
Australia	School and studying mean very little to me.	22	26	14	22
Germany	School and education mean very little to me.	9	6	9	9
Italy	School/studying have very little value for me.	18	17	13	11
Israel	School and studies are not important to me.	28	27	18	16
Hungary	School and studying mean very little to me.	16	30	12	18
Turkey	School and studying mean very little to me.	36	34	28	24
Japan	Schoolwork is not important to me.	—	10	—	8
Taiwan	School and studying mean little to me.	18	14	11	13
Bangladesh	School and studying have very little meaning for me.	40	31	21	15

Sexual Self (SxS)
SCALE: SEXUAL ATTITUDES

---

10. The opposite sex finds me a bore. (−)

28. Dirty jokes are fun at times.

77. I think that girls/boys find me attractive

80. I do not attend sexy shows. (−)

91. Sexually I am way behind. (−)

97. Thinking or talking about sex scares me. (−)

117. Sexual experiences give me pleasure.

119. Having a girl-/boyfriend is important to me.

122. I often think about sex.

ITEM 10

Country	Translation	YM	OM	YF	OF
United States	The opposite sex finds me a bore.	18	11	13	9
Australia	The opposite sex finds me a bore.	19	15	22	12
Germany	The opposite sex finds me boring.	6	10	10	7
Italy	The opposite sex considers me a bore.	11	5	8	7
Israel	The opposite sex thinks I am boring.	22	22	11	9
Hungary	Members of the opposite sex usually find me boring.	12	13	10	9
Turkey	The opposite sex finds me boring.	22	13	18	11
Japan	People of the opposite sex find me boring.	—	38	—	38
Taiwan	I am considered not interesting by the opposite sex.	21	18	13	14
Bangladesh	The opposite sex does not like my company.	30	29	27	18

ITEM 28

Country	Translation	YM	OM	YF	OF
United States	Dirty jokes are fun at times.	80	84	74	75
Australia	Dirty jokes are fun at times.	81	87	79	81
Germany	Dirty jokes are sometimes funny.	77	69	66	62
Italy	Sometimes dirty (risqué) jokes are entertaining.	76	83	56	62
Israel	Dirty jokes are funny at times.	85	81	77	69
Hungary	Sometimes I enjoy dirty jokes.	42	63	24	27
Turkey	Dirty jokes can sometimes be amusing.	28	33	8	5
Japan	Dirty jokes and stories are sometimes funny.	—	87	—	83
Taiwan	Sometimes, cheap jokes are interesting.	51	71	29	21
Bangladesh	Sometimes even dirty jokes amuse me.	33	45	23	32

ITEM 77

Country	Translation	YM	OM	YF	OF
United States	I think that girls/boys find me attractive.	72	79	71	69
Australia	I think that girls/boys find me attractive.	62	66	40	42
Germany	I think that girls/boys find me attractive.	59	69	53	70
Italy	I believe that girls/boys find me attractive.	65	63	41	49
Israel	It seems to me that girls/boys think I am attractive.	69	63	75	65
Hungary	I feel members of the opposite sex find me attractive.	58	58	56	60
Turkey	I think that girls/boys find me attractive.	59	69	42	64
Japan	I am sure girls/boys find me attractive.	—	17	—	6
Taiwan	I think the opposite sex finds me attractive.	38	61	20	43
Bangladesh	I think that girls/boys find me attractive.	56	69	68	60

ITEM 80

Country	Translation	YM	OM	YF	OF
United States	I do not attend sexy shows.	41	48	68	60
Australia	I do not attend sexy shows.	36	40	55	55
Germany	I don't go to sex shows.	59	80	72	86
Italy	I never go to pornos.	27	33	74	72
Israel	I don't go to X-rated movies and shows.	44	54	68	73
Hungary	I would not watch a show that only showed sex.	22	17	47	35
Turkey	I don't go to sexually arousing (sexy) shows.	55	44	71	70
Japan	I will not see a sex-exploited show.	—	62	—	79
Taiwan	I will not see sex shows.	64	33	73	70
Bangladesh	I do not like looking at (erotic) (sexual) pictures.	61	48	60	75

ITEM 91

Country	Translation	YM	OM	YF	OF
United States	Sexually I am way behind.	18	21	26	32
Australia	Sexually I am way behind.	12	17	26	25
Germany	Sexually I am somehow behind.	10	9	13	11
Italy	I am sexually retarded.	5	3	13	8
Israel	I am sexually retarded.	7	11	12	8
Hungary	I am sexually underdeveloped.	10	10	13	12
Turkey	Sexually I am very behind.	19	8	21	28
Japan	I am sexually behind others.	—	24	—	29
Taiwan	I am behind in sexual matters.	24	27	42	39
Bangladesh	There is a lack of sexual passion in me.	29	25	31	17

ITEM 97

Country	Translation	YM	OM	YF	OF
United States	Thinking or talking about sex scares me.	16	2	13	7
Australia	Thinking or talking about sex scares me.	6	4	13	5
Germany	Thinking or talking about sex makes me anxious.	8	3	8	5
Italy	I am afraid to think or talk about sexual topics.	7	4	13	5
Israel	Thoughts or talking about sex scares me.	5	6	9	5
Hungary	I am afraid to think or talk about sex.	15	9	17	9
Turkey	I am afraid to think or talk about sexuality (topics relating to sex).	23	12	36	18
Japan	I am afraid to think and talk about sex.	—	7	—	10
Taiwan	Thinking or talking about sex frightens me.	27	17	36	28
Bangladesh	I fear thinking or talking about sexual matters.	48	37	71	45

ITEM 117

Country	Translation	YM	OM	YF	OF
United States	Sexual experiences give me pleasure.	83	88	53	70
Australia	Sexual experiences give me pleasure.	75	85	43	63
Germany	Sexual experiences give me pleasure.	72	80	44	71
Italy	Sexual experiences are pleasing to me.	80	88	34	66
Israel	I find sexual experiences pleasurable.	84	89	52	61
Hungary	Sexual experiences give me pleasure.	69	86	39	66
Turkey	I enjoy sexual experience.	60	85	19	33
Japan	Sex is a pleasurable experience.	—	75	—	32
Taiwan	Sexual experiences bring me pleasure.	26	40	13	7
Bangladesh	I am happy to acquire sexual knowledge.	42	59	30	44

ITEM 119

Country	Translation	YM	OM	YF	OF
United States	Having a girl-/boyfriend is important to me.	79	72	66	75
Australia	Having a girl-/boyfriend is important to me.	78	75	60	62
Germany	It is important for me to have a friend.	83	91	73	80
Italy	To have a girlfriend (boyfriend) is very important to me.	82	80	73	70
Israel	It is important to have a girl-/boyfriend.	79	75	72	75
Hungary	It is important to me to have a girl/boy to go out with.	69	78	52	72
Turkey	It is important for me to have a girl-/boyfriend.	68	82	66	78
Japan	To me it is important to have a girl-/boyfriend.	—	75	—	70
Taiwan	It is important for me to have a good friend of the opposite sex.	61	74	29	45
Bangladesh	I need to have a girl/boy friend.	71	80	72	85

ITEM 122

Country	Translation	YM	OM	YF	OF
United States	I often think about sex.	69	71	55	59
Australia	I often think about sex.	73	78	40	54
Germany	I often think about sex.	62	60	38	42
Italy	I think frequently about sex.	72	65	32	38
Israel	I often think about sex.	74	78	54	45
Hungary	I often think about sex.	58	71	25	37
Turkey	I think about sexual topics often.	49	58	28	32
Japan	I think about sex often.	—	71	—	57
Taiwan	I often think about sexual matters.	35	67	27	25
Bangladesh	I often think about sexual things.	28	45	20	27

4. I think that I will be a source of pride to my parents in the future.

9. My parents are almost always on the side of someone else, e.g., my brother or sister. (−)

15. My parents will be disappointed in me in the future. (−)

21. Very often I feel that my father is no good. (−)

24. Understanding my parents is beyond me. (−)

51. Most of the time my parents get along well with each other.

55. When my parents are strict, I feel that they are right, even if I get angry.

60. When I grow up and have a family, it will be in at least a few ways similar to my own.

64. I feel that I have a part in making family decisions.

71. My parents are usually patient with me.

73. Very often parents do not understand a person because they had an unhappy childhood. (−)

85. Usually I feel that I am a bother at home. (−)

87. I like one of my parents much better than the other. (−)

95. My parents are ashamed of me. (−)

102. I try to stay away from home most of the time. (−)

106. I have been carrying a grudge against my parents for years. (−)

112. Most of the time my parents are satisfied with me.

118. Very often I feel that my mother is no good. (−)

ITEM 4

Country	Translation	YM	OM	YF	OF
United States	I think that I will be a source of pride to my parents in the future.	90	92	90	84
Australia	I think that I will be a source of pride to my parents in the future.	77	76	73	60
Germany	I believe that in the future I will be a source of joy for my parents.	59	60	61	59
Italy	I believe that in the future my parents will be proud of me.	81	77	78	70
Israel	I think that in the future I will be a source of pride for my parents.	84	86	84	81
Hungary	I believe my parents will be proud of me eventually.	63	58	60	56
Turkey	I think (believe) that I will be a source of pride for my mother and father in the future.	81	82	79	84
Japan	My parents will be proud of my accomplishments.	—	29	—	23
Taiwan	I think my parents will be proud of me.	73	78	47	82
Bangladesh	I think my parents will be proud of me in the future.	81	91	91	82

ITEM 9

Country	Translation	YM	OM	YF	OF
United States	My parents are almost always on the side of someone else, e.g., my brother or sister.	30	29	32	25
Australia	My parents are almost always on the side of someone else, e.g., my brother or sister.	51	40	50	42
Germany	My parents almost always take someone else's side, for example my brother's or my sister's.	15	10	15	12
Italy	My parents always worry about somebody else, such as my brother or sister.	19	11	33	20
Israel	My parents side with someone else almost always, for example my brother or my sister.	29	14	28	15
Hungary	My parents generally take someone else's side (e.g., my brother's or sister's).	31	30	18	16
Turkey	My parents often show preference for someone else, like my brother or my sister.	23	18	22	15
Japan	Frequently, my parents take sides with my siblings against me.	—	17	—	18
Taiwan	My parents often stand on other people's side, e.g., my brother or sister.	35	8	27	13
Bangladesh	My parents frequently side with others, that is side with my brother or sister.	33	30	38	39

ITEM 15

Country	Translation	YM	OM	YF	OF
United States	My parents will be disappointed in me in the future.	9	3	7	7
Australia	My parents will be disappointed in me in the future.	16	15	10	11
Germany	My parents will be disappointed with me in the future.	3	7	8	6
Italy	My parents will not be proud of me in the future.	9	5	10	6
Israel	My parents will be disappointed by me in the future.	7	8	7	3
Hungary	My parents will be disappointed in me.	8	16	4	6
Turkey	I will be a source of disappointment for my mother and father.	17	10	16	10
Japan	My parents will probably be disappointed in me in the future.	—	27	—	21
Taiwan	In the future, my parents will be disappointed in me.	27	16	22	23
Bangladesh	My parents will be disappointed in me in the future.	12	9	9	12

ITEM 21

Country	Translation	YM	OM	YF	OF
United States	Very often I feel that my father is no good.	15	10	22	13
Australia	Very often I feel that my father is no good.	18	14	21	24
Germany	I very often feel that my father is no good.	3	10	13	11
Italy	Quite often I believe that my father hasn't been a good one.	12	14	18	15
Israel	I often feel like a failure.	7	5	5	8
Hungary	I feel very often that my father is not a good man.	8	15	12	18
Turkey	I often feel my father is good for nothing (worthless).	7	9	7	8
Japan	Often I find it difficult to find my father's good points.	—	13	—	15
Taiwan	I often feel that my father is not good enough.	20	19	11	22
Bangladesh	I frequently think that my father is ineffective.	12	13	11	12

ITEM 24

Country	Translation	YM	OM	YF	OF
United States	Understanding my parents is beyond me.	20	13	15	17
Australia	Understanding my parents is beyond me.	29	15	30	30
Germany	I just can't succeed in understanding my parents.	9	9	20	10
Italy	Understanding my parents is over and above what I can endure (do).	11	6	18	12
Israel	I can't understand my parents.	20	18	21	17
Hungary	I am unable to understand my parents.	10	18	9	11
Turkey	To understand my mother and father is beyond me.	22	15	29	19
Japan	It is hard for me to understand my parents.	—	15	—	24
Taiwan	I have difficulties understanding my parents.	29	15	22	24
Bangladesh	It is beyond my powers to understand my parents.	27	26	25	21

ITEM 51

Country	Translation	YM	OM	YF	OF
United States	Most of the time my parents get along well with each other.	84	76	79	72
Australia	Most of the time my parents get along well with each other.	85	83	79	70
Germany	Most of the time my parents get along well with one another.	85	71	76	69
Italy	Usually my parents get along well.	88	81	80	75
Israel	Most of the time my parents get along well.	88	87	82	83
Hungary	My parents usually get along well.	81	80	80	70
Turkey	My mother and father get along well most of the time.	92	87	89	89
Japan	Usually my parents are happy together.	—	77	—	81
Taiwan	Most of the time, my parents get along well.	94	82	98	72
Bangladesh	My parents maintain a good relationship between them most of the time.	87	88	88	86

ITEM 55

Country	Translation	YM	OM	YF	OF
United States	When my parents are strict, I feel that they are right, even if I get angry.	59	65	55	65
Australia	When my parents are strict, I feel that they are right, even if I get angry.	70	60	57	56
Germany	When my parents are strict, I feel they are right even if I get angry about it.	50	34	41	26
Italy	When my parents are tough I believe they are right even if I get mad.	79	64	73	57
Israel	When my parents are strict with me, I think they are right even if it angers me.	37	42	42	42
Hungary	When my parents are strict, I feel they are right even if I complain about it.	69	54	75	56
Turkey	When my mother and father get tough, I feel they are right even if I am angry with them.	69	76	67	73
Japan	When my parents get angry at me and I get mad—I still believe they are right.	—	35	—	31
Taiwan	Even though I am angry at my parents' strictness, I think they are right.	91	73	71	64
Bangladesh	When my parents are harsh to me I feel angry but I still think that they are blameless.	83	87	91	81

ITEM 60

Country	Translation	YM	OM	YF	OF
United States	When I grow up and have a family, it will be in at least a few ways similar to my own.	82	86	74	80
Australia	When I grow up and have a family, it will be in at least a few ways similar to my own.	57	69	62	52
Germany	When I grow up and have a family, it will be like my own in at least a few things.	59	67	59	57
Italy	When I grow up and establish a family it will be somewhat similar to my present family.	74	62	63	59
Israel	When I grow up and have a family, it will be similar to mine in some aspect.	76	78	76	73
Hungary	When I have a family, in at least a few respects it will be like my current one.	79	68	76	73
Turkey	When I grow up and have a family, it will be similar to my family in at least a few respects.	77	81	70	68
Japan	When I have my own family, it will have some qualities of the family I am a part of today.	—	80	—	83
Taiwan	When I grow up and have a family, it will be similar to my family at least in some ways.	76	74	75	59
Bangladesh	When I grow up and have a family, that will be at least like the present one.	50	48	58	37

ITEM 64

Country	Translation	YM	OM	YF	OF
United States	I feel that I have a part in making family decisions.	72	74	71	68
Australia	I feel that I have a part in making family decisions.	61	79	64	67
Germany	I have the feeling of participating in family decisions.	80	76	68	83
Italy	I feel like I have a part in the decision making of my family.	73	75	71	72
Israel	I feel that I participate in decision making in my family.	78	75	83	79
Hungary	I feel that I can take part in family decisions.	78	80	86	87
Turkey	I feel that I have a part in the decisions made in the family.	60	85	67	87
Japan	I believe I am part of most family decisions.	—	70	—	79
Taiwan	I feel that I always have a part in making family decisions.	66	67	62	67
Bangladesh	I think that I have a role in family decisions.	87	80	92	96

ITEM 71

Country	Translation	YM	OM	YF	OF
United States	My parents are usually patient with me.	82	88	81	83
Australia	My parents are usually patient with me.	62	79	65	67
Germany	My parents are usually patient with me.	86	82	72	78
Italy	My parents are patient with me.	84	80	79	77
Israel	My parents generally treat me with patience.	92	92	89	90
Hungary	My parents are usually patient with me.	84	79	87	79
Turkey	My mother and father are usually patient toward me.	83	88	80	80
Japan	My parents are patient with me.	—	75	—	72
Taiwan	My parents can usually tolerate me.	73	88	69	84
Bangladesh	My parents are usually patient with me.	87	88	95	91

ITEM 73

Country	Translation	YM	OM	YF	OF
United States	Very often parents do not understand a person because they had an unhappy childhood.	28	23	22	27
Australia	Very often parents do not understand a person because they had an unhappy childhood.	49	36	39	30
Germany	Very often parents don't understand someone else because they had an unhappy childhood.	33	38	29	34
Italy	My parents frequently don't understand a person because they had an unhappy infancy.	30	23	31	29
Israel	Often my parents don't understand others because they suffered in their childhood.	27	22	16	16
Hungary	Parents often misunderstand because they had an unhappy childhood.	26	28	20	20
Turkey	Parents usually do not understand people because they passed unhappy childhoods.	32	27	42	34
Japan	My parents cannot understand and relate with others because of their unhappy childhood.	—	25	—	19
Taiwan	Because parents have unhappy childhoods, therefore they usually cannot understand me.	18	16	11	16
Bangladesh	My parents were unhappy as children, perhaps that is why they do not wish to properly understand anyone.	21	26	15	21

ITEM 85

Country	Translation	YM	OM	YF	OF
United States	Usually I feel that I am a bother at home.	24	17	22	19
Australia	Usually I feel that I am a bother at home.	35	34	43	34
Germany	At home I usually have the feeling of getting on other people's nerves.	23	16	24	13
Italy	At home I usually feel that I am a burden to the family.	11	5	16	9
Israel	Generally I feel that I am a nuisance at home.	10	10	7	8
Hungary	I often feel that I am just a bother at home.	10	16	9	10
Turkey	Most of the time I feel that I am a problem.	41	33	39	26
Japan	Usually I feel that I am a bothersome figure in my family.	—	22	—	21
Taiwan	I often feel that I am not liked at home.	22	9	20	11
Bangladesh	I usually feel that I am an irritating person at home.	16	18	14	16

ITEM 87

Country	Translation	YM	OM	YF	OF
United States	I like one of my parents much better than the other.	22	24	32	34
Australia	I like one of my parents much better than the other.	21	15	35	32
Germany	I like one of my parents a lot more than the other.	31	23	30	25
Italy	I like one of my parents much more than the other.	15	15	25	26
Israel	I love one of my parents much more than the other.	19	14	14	20
Hungary	I like one of my parents much better than the other.	12	24	18	21
Turkey	I like one of my parents more than the other.	24	21	24	25
Japan	I have a certain attraction to one of my parents over the other.	—	34	—	53
Taiwan	I like one of my parents better than the other.	44	38	33	44
Bangladesh	I love one of my parents more than the other.	38	34	48	34

ITEM 95

Country	Translation	YM	OM	YF	OF
United States	My parents are ashamed of me.	10	5	7	5
Australia	My parents are ashamed of me.	9	13	10	11
Germany	My parents are ashamed of me.	3	1	3	1
Italy	My parents are ashamed of me.	5	3	6	1
Israel	My parents are ashamed of me.	2	4	4	1
Hungary	My parents are ashamed of me.	5	6	2	4
Turkey	My parents are ashamed of me.	12	7	9	2
Japan	My parents are embarrassed of me.	—	14	—	15
Taiwan	My parents are ashamed of me.	16	6	13	6
Bangladesh	My parents are ashamed of me.	9	8	6	5

ITEM 102

Country	Translation	YM	OM	YF	OF
United States	I try to stay away from home most of the time.	23	21	25	23
Australia	I try to stay away from home most of the time.	26	21	22	23
Germany	I try to be mostly away from home.	18	25	29	26
Italy	I try to stay outside home as much as I can.	38	35	38	31
Israel	I try to be out of the house most of the time.	31	36	34	25
Hungary	I try to get away from home as much as possible.	18	34	13	23
Turkey	Most of the time I try to stay away from home.	34	37	35	37
Japan	Usually I try to stay away from home.	—	14	—	11
Taiwan	I often want to stay out and not to go home.	26	29	24	14
Bangladesh	I try to spend most of my time outside my house.	39	32	26	22

ITEM 106

Country	Translation	YM	OM	YF	OF
United States	I have been carrying a grudge against my parents for years.	9	11	14	12
Australia	I have been carrying a grudge against my parents for years.	8	11	13	20
Germany	For years, I have harbored resentment against my parents.	1	3	5	6
Italy	I have a grudge with my parents for many years.	6	3	7	3
Israel	I have resented my parents for years.	6	6	6	5
Hungary	I have been carrying a grudge against my parents for years.	7	13	6	10
Turkey	For years I have nurtured a grudge against my parents.	3	4	7	3
Japan	I have a grudge against my parents.	—	8	—	15
Taiwan	I have strong disapproval/dissatisfaction of my parents for years.	13	14	16	17
Bangladesh	I have been carrying around a grudge against my parents for a long time.	14	11	16	19

ITEM 112

Country	Translation	YM	OM	YF	OF
United States	Most of the time my parents are satisfied with me.	86	89	80	84
Australia	Most of the time my parents are satisfied with me.	87	85	82	79
Germany	Most of the time my parents are satisfied with me.	90	76	74	75
Italy	Usually my parents are satisfied with me.	78	81	77	79
Israel	Most of the time my parents are satisfied with me.	89	87	86	86
Hungary	My parents are generally satisfied with me.	84	67	84	78
Turkey	Mostly my mother and father are pleased with me.	81	90	90	89
Japan	Usually my parents are satisfied with me.	—	59	—	55
Taiwan	Most of the time, my parents are satisfied/happy with me.	75	79	67	78
Bangladesh	My parents are not satisfied with me most of the time.	89	75	86	85

ITEM 118

Country	Translation	YM	OM	YF	OF
United States	Very often I feel that my mother is no good.	13	12	14	11
Australia	Very often I feel that my mother is no good.	8	8	15	11
Germany	Very often I have the feeling that my mother is no good.	5	5	9	2
Italy	Frequently I feel that my mother has not been a good mother.	8	5	10	9
Israel	Often I feel that my mother is worthless.	9	9	11	6
Hungary	I often feel my mother is not a good person.	7	11	5	11
Turkey	I feel very often that my mother is worthless.	8	8	2	3
Japan	Often I feel there are no good qualities in my mother.	—	16	—	18
Taiwan	I often feel my mother is not good enough.	13	17	13	16
Bangladesh	It often seems to me that my mother is quite useless (ineffective).	14	11	6	9

19. If I put my mind to it, I can learn almost anything.
76. When I decide to do something, I do it.
103. I find life an endless series of problems—without solution in sight. (−)
105. I feel that I am able to make decisions.
109. I feel that I have no talent whatsoever. (−)

ITEM 19

Country	Translation	YM	OM	YF	OF
United States	If I put my mind to it, I can learn almost anything.	91	93	93	89
Australia	If I put my mind to it, I can learn almost anything.	90	87	86	81
Germany	When I try hard, I can learn almost anything.	77	74	71	76
Italy	I really think I can learn almost anything.	81	81	86	79
Israel	When I try hard, I can learn almost anything.	96	93	95	96
Hungary	If I make up my mind I can learn anything.	85	85	87	87
Turkey	If I set my mind to it I can learn everything.	91	94	89	94
Japan	If I concentrate and work hard I can learn anything.	—	69	—	67
Taiwan	If I put my mind to it, I can learn everything.	91	81	84	84
Bangladesh	If I try attentively I can learn anything.	98	100	96	99

ITEM 76

Country	Translation	YM	OM	YF	OF
United States	When I decide to do something, I do it.	80	85	88	89
Australia	When I decide to do something, I do it.	76	79	73	78
Germany	When I make a decision to do something, I do it.	82	84	81	86
Italy	When I decide to do something, I do it.	76	75	71	75
Israel	When I decide to do something, I do it.	87	78	86	84
Hungary	If I decide something, I do it.	85	84	83	85
Turkey	When I decide on doing something, I do it.	83	90	83	92
Japan	When I decide to do something, I do it.	—	77	—	81
Taiwan	When I decide to do something, I do it.	76	66	51	60
Bangladesh	When I decide to do something, I usually accomplish it.	78	86	86	78

ITEM 103

Country	Translation	YM	OM	YF	OF
United States	I find life an endless series of problems—without solution in sight.	20	10	14	16
Australia	I find life an endless series of problems—without solution in sight.	30	28	28	22
Germany	In my opinion life is an endless series of unsolvable problems.	24	13	19	16
Italy	I find that life is an endless series of problems without any solutions in sight.	16	12	13	11
Israel	Life seems to be endless series of problems without solutions.	23	26	25	17
Hungary	For me life is full of problems without solutions.	6	15	7	14
Turkey	I see life as an infinite (endless) series of problems without any solutions.	36	33	41	36
Japan	I feel there is no end to life and all of its challenges.	—	44	—	34
Taiwan	I find that life is a series of unending problems—with no ways to find solutions.	20	38	32	33
Bangladesh	In life I find only endless problems for which I can find no solution.	36	37	36	46

ITEM 105

Country	Translation	YM	OM	YF	OF
United States	I feel that I am able to make decisions.	89	89	87	93
Australia	I feel that I am able to make decisions.	86	83	72	83
Germany	I believe I can make decisions.	90	97	82	91
Italy	I feel like I can make decisions.	81	83	73	76
Israel	I feel that I can make decisions.	92	94	95	94
Hungary	I feel I can make decisions.	88	87	83	84
Turkey	I feel that I am competent to make decisions.	74	89	69	80
Japan	I feel I am capable of making various decisions.	—	51	—	45
Taiwan	I feel that I have the ability to make decisions.	76	82	73	77
Bangladesh	I have the power to make decisions.	90	90	86	86

ITEM 109

Country	Translation	YM	OM	YF	OF
United States	I feel that I have no talent whatsoever.	13	6	11	11
Australia	I feel that I have no talent whatsoever.	15	10	19	16
Germany	I believe I don't have any talent at all.	5	5	14	6
Italy	I feel I do not have any talent.	43	6	71	9
Israel	I feel that I lack talent altogether.	4	5	8	8
Hungary	I feel I have no talent for anything.	6	11	8	12
Turkey	I feel that I don't have any talent at all.	19	12	21	16
Japan	I have absolutely no talent.	—	32	—	39
Taiwan	I feel that I have no talent in any area.	31	23	27	29
Bangladesh	I do not believe that I have any talent.	26	24	21	15

Coping Self (CS-2)
SCALE: PSYCHOPATHOLOGY

---

2. When I am with people, I am afraid that someone will make fun of me. (−)

22. I am confused most of the time. (−)

29. I often blame myself even when I am not at fault. (−)

31. The size of my sex organs is normal.

36. Sometimes I feel so ashamed of myself that I just want to hide in a corner and cry. (−)

45. I feel empty emotionally most of the time. (−)

61. I often feel that I would rather die than go on living. (−)

93. Even though I am continuously on the go, I seem unable to get things done. (−)

96. I believe I can tell the real from the fantastic.

126. I do not have many fears which I cannot understand.

ITEM 2

Country	Translation	YM	OM	YF	OF
United States	When I am with people, I am afraid that someone will make fun of me.	20	17	28	25
Australia	When I am with people, I am afraid that someone will make fun of me.	32	20	31	20
Germany	When I am with people, I am very worried that someone is going to make fun of me.	5	14	17	16
Italy	When I am with people, I am afraid that somebody is making jokes about me.	25	20	36	35
Israel	When I am with other people, I am afraid of someone mocking me.	26	19	22	18
Hungary	When I am with others, I am afraid they are making fun of me.	6	9	11	13
Turkey	When I am with other people, I am afraid that someone is going to make fun of me.	39	34	43	29
Japan	I am often afraid of being mocked within a large crowd.	—	22	—	21
Taiwan	When I am with other people, I am afraid someone will make fun of me.	47	36	33	24
Bangladesh	When I am among people, I fear that someone may make fun of me.	29	23	37	27

ITEM 22

Country	Translation	YM	OM	YF	OF
United States	I am confused most of the time.	16	10	22	19
Australia	I am confused most of the time.	13	16	24	22
Germany	Most of the time I am confused.	8	6	14	7
Italy	I often feel confused.	13	13	30	26
Israel	Most of the time I am confused.	6	10	17	16
Hungary	I am often scattered.	27	39	25	34
Turkey	Most of the time my mind is confused (mixed up).	47	43	54	45
Japan	I am frequently rushed and confused.	—	55	—	66
Taiwan	I often feel confused.	46	48	51	65
Bangladesh	Most of the time I confuse everything.	31	42	51	54

ITEM 29

Country	Translation	YM	OM	YF	OF
United States	I often blame myself even when I am not at fault.	34	41	36	34
Australia	I often blame myself even when I am not at fault.	36	40	39	45
Germany	I often blame myself even when I haven't done anything wrong.	17	31	26	26
Italy	Often I reprimand myself even when I am not guilty.	39	38	42	41
Israel	Often I blame myself, even when I am not guilty.	22	27	26	29
Hungary	I often feel guilty even when it is not my fault.	21	23	23	31
Turkey	Even if I am not guilty, very often I hold (feel) myself guilty.	36	32	32	36
Japan	Even if I am not guilty I will still take the blame.	—	34	—	34
Taiwan	Even if it is not my fault, I often blame myself.	38	46	49	53
Bangladesh	I frequently accuse myself needlessly.	43	46	43	53

ITEM 31

Country	Translation	YM	OM	YF	OF
United States	The size of my sex organs is normal.	91	88	92	93
Australia	The size of my sex organs is normal.	92	91	91	91
Germany	My sex organs are normal.	96	96	100	99
Italy	My sex organs are normal.	97	96	97	97
Israel	My genitals are of normal size.	93	93	97	93
Hungary	The size of my sexual organ is normal.	88	90	93	90
Turkey	The size of my genitals (sex organs) are normal.	71	91	58	85
Japan	My genitals are of average size.	—	83	—	87
Taiwan	The size of my sex organ is normal.	93	89	82	81
Bangladesh	The shape/size of my sexual organs is normal.	87	85	89	90

ITEM 36

Country	Translation	YM	OM	YF	OF
United States	Sometimes I feel so ashamed of myself that I just want to hide in a corner and cry.	22	17	37	23
Australia	Sometimes I feel so ashamed of myself that I just want to hide in a corner and cry.	24	15	39	41
Germany	Sometimes I feel so embarrassed that I feel like hiding in a corner and crying.	14	7	27	18
Italy	At times I am so ashamed I would like to hide.	21	12	35	21
Israel	At times I am so ashamed of myself that I feel like hiding in a corner and crying.	27	18	29	27
Hungary	Sometimes I am so ashamed that I would prefer to hide somewhere and just cry.	16	11	26	26
Turkey	Sometimes I feel so ashamed (embarrassed) of myself, I want to hide in a corner and cry.	28	20	26	23
Japan	Sometimes I am embarrassed and want to hide in a corner and cry.	—	28	—	47
Taiwan	Sometimes I feel ashamed and only want to hide and cry in a corner.	26	23	38	41
Bangladesh	Sometimes I feel so ashamed of myself that I wish to hide in a corner and weep.	32	35	31	27

ITEM 45

Country	Translation	YM	OM	YF	OF
United States	I feel empty emotionally most of the time.	26	16	14	17
Australia	I feel empty emotionally most of the time.	31	22	27	27
Germany	Most of the time I don't feel anything.	17	8	3	2
Italy	Usually I feel empty emotionally.	27	27	30	30
Israel	Most of the time I feel emotional emptiness.	23	19	17	21
Hungary	I feel emotionally empty most of the time.	13	18	8	7
Turkey	I feel emotionally drained (empty) most of the time.	41	42	39	46
Japan	Usually I feel empty in life.	—	26	—	32
Taiwan	I often feel empty.	33	53	44	56
Bangladesh	Mentally, most of the time, I feel empty of emotions.	41	36	36	41

ITEM 61

Country	Translation	YM	OM	YF	OF
United States	I often feel that I would rather die than go on living.	15	16	26	18
Australia	I often feel that I would rather die than go on living.	28	26	34	30
Germany	I often feel that I would rather die than live anymore.	21	13	25	18
Italy	I often think that it is better to die than live.	15	9	22	13
Israel	Frequently I feel like dying rather than going on and living.	16	12	24	22
Hungary	I often feel that I would rather die than keep on living.	13	17	15	21
Turkey	Often I feel that I would rather die than go on living.	25	18	28	27
Japan	I sometimes feel that I would rather be dead than alive.	—	21	—	18
Taiwan	I often feel that I would rather be dead than alive.	13	10	16	16
Bangladesh	I often think that it is better for me to die than to live.	29	28	48	47

ITEM 93

Country	Translation	YM	OM	YF	OF
United States	Even though I am continuously on the go, I seem unable to get things done.	40	31	29	29
Australia	Even though I am continuously on the go, I seem unable to get things done.	28	35	34	36
Germany	Even though I try constantly, I seem to be incapable of finishing things.	22	7	15	5
Italy	Even if I am constantly trying, it looks as though I am unable to go finish anything.	21	14	27	20
Israel	Even though I'm busy all the time, I can't complete things.	27	26	21	22
Hungary	Despite the fact that I am always trying, I cannot get things done.	17	24	15	18
Turkey	I am continually active, however I can't finish my work.	48	29	34	27
Japan	Even though I am very active I accomplish very little.	—	42	—	38
Taiwan	Although I continue to do things, I have not accomplished anything.	43	45	36	56
Bangladesh	Even though I work at all times, yet it seems to me that I am unable to complete the work.	42	30	46	50

ITEM 96

Country	Translation	YM	OM	YF	OF
United States	I believe I can tell the real from the fantastic.	84	89	83	82
Australia	I believe I can tell the real from the fantastic.	69	78	65	71
Germany	I believe I can distinguish fantasy from reality.	82	94	76	82
Italy	I am convinced that I cannot distinguish reality from fantasy.	78	77	70	64
Israel	I believe I can differentiate reality from fantasy.	95	87	89	89
Hungary	I believe I can distinguish reality from fantasy.	84	87	86	89
Turkey	I believe I can discern between reality and fantasy.	76	90	78	92
Japan	I believe I can separate fantasy and reality.	—	80	—	77
Taiwan	I believe I can differentiate facts from fancy.	93	83	80	78
Bangladesh	I believe I can give something imagined the form of a true story.	66	68	69	49

ITEM 126

Country	Translation	YM	OM	YF	OF
United States	I do not have many fears which I cannot understand.	68	90	76	72
Australia	I do not have many fears which I cannot understand.	64	79	69	70
Germany	I do not have many fears that I can't understand.	47	81	51	68
Italy	I usually am not afraid of things I cannot understand.	57	63	55	53
Israel	I don't have many fears that I cannot understand.	76	81	81	77
Hungary	I do not have many inexplicable fears.	73	74	72	72
Turkey	I don't have many fears that I cannot understand.	70	78	71	69
Japan	I do not have many fears that I cannot understand.	—	66	—	62
Taiwan	I am not too afraid of things I cannot understand.	82	79	69	73
Bangladesh	I am not often needlessly frightened.	61	67	75	80

Coping Self (CS-3)
SCALE: SUPERIOR ADJUSTMENT

---

25. I do not like to put things in order and make sense of them. (−)

39. When a tragedy occurs to one of my friends, I feel sad too.

49. Our society is a competitive one and I am not afraid of it.

53. I find it very difficult to establish new friendships. (−)

56. Working closely with another fellow never gives me pleasure (−)

84. If I know that I will have to face a new situation, I will try in advance to find out as much as is possible about it.

89. Whenever I fail in something, I try to find out what I can do in order to avoid another failure.

107. I am certain that I will not be able to assume responsibilities for myself in the future. (−)

110. I do not rehearse how I might deal with a real coming event. (−)

114. I do not enjoy solving difficult problems. (−)

121. Worrying a little about one's future helps to make it work out better.

ITEM 25

Country	Translation	YM	OM	YF	OF
United States	I do not like to put things in order and make sense of them.	13	8	10	7
Australia	I do not like to put things in order and make sense of them.	19	19	22	7
Germany	I don't enjoy putting things in order and understanding their meaning.	14	13	25	9
Italy	I don't particularly like trying to make sense out of everything.	25	19	25	16
Israel	I don't like to order things logically.	22	15	10	10
Hungary	I don't like to keep things in order, and I don't see the point of doing it.	17	30	12	13
Turkey	I don't like to put things in order and make sense out of it.	47	31	41	40
Japan	I do not like to have everything neat and organized.	—	31	—	20
Taiwan	I do not like to do things in a proper and orderly manner, or to make them meaningful.	26	22	22	22
Bangladesh	I do not like to keep things neatly organized.	25	20	10	10

ITEM 39

Country	Translation	YM	OM	YF	OF
United States	When a tragedy occurs to one of my friends, I feel sad too.	88	93	93	97
Australia	When a tragedy occurs to one of my friends, I feel sad too.	85	80	95	91
Germany	If something bad happens to a friend of mine I feel sad, too.	72	86	98	97
Italy	When something sad befalls my friend, I feel sad myself.	85	87	93	93
Israel	When a friend of mine goes through a tragedy, I too feel sad.	88	85	91	92
Hungary	If a friend were to suffer a terrible mishap, I would also be sad.	78	76	89	95
Turkey	If something real bad should happen to one of my friends, I would also feel sorry (bad).	89	92	96	96
Japan	If something sad happens to my friends I too become sad.	—	62	—	89
Taiwan	When a tragedy occurs to one of my friends, I feel sad too.	84	94	96	93
Bangladesh	If something sad happens in the life of one of my friends, I too feel sad.	89	91	95	97

ITEM 49

Country	Translation	YM	OM	YF	OF
United States	Our society is a competitive one and I am not afraid of it.	78	75	65	71
Australia	Our society is a competitive one and I am not afraid of it.	68	74	58	56
Germany	Our society is founded on competition and I am not afraid of it.	64	66	34	32
Italy	Society is competitive, and I am not afraid of it.	52	56	41	35
Israel	Our society is competitive, and I am not afraid of it.	72	70	64	53
Hungary	Our society is competitive, and I am not afraid of this competition.	67	60	66	48
Turkey	Our society is very competitive, and I am not afraid of it.	63	74	63	69
Japan	I am not afraid of this competitive society.	—	52	—	49
Taiwan	We are a competitive society, but I am not afraid of it.	71	78	58	68
Bangladesh	Our society is competitive, but that does not frighten me.	82	87	85	85

ITEM 53

Country	Translation	YM	OM	YF	OF
United States	I find it very difficult to establish new friendships.	28	21	17	18
Australia	I find it very difficult to establish new friendships.	31	23	22	21
Germany	I find it very hard to make new friends.	22	23	24	24
Italy	It is very hard for me to make new friends.	26	26	28	25
Israel	I find it hard to establish new friendships.	27	30	18	24
Hungary	It is difficult for me to initiate friendships.	22	30	17	32
Turkey	I find it very difficult to establish new relationships (friendships).	33	32	33	30
Japan	It is very hard for me to make new friends.	—	43	—	39
Taiwan	I think it is very difficult to build new friendships.	30	29	20	29
Bangladesh	It seems very difficult for me to establish new friendships.	51	39	41	38

ITEM 56

Country	Translation	YM	OM	YF	OF
United States	Working closely with another fellow never gives me pleasure.	34	31	26	20
Australia	Working closely with another fellow never gives me pleasure.	39	38	19	20
Germany	I never enjoy working closely with a boy/girl friend.	21	14	13	7
Italy	I don't like to work in close collaboration with another boy/girl.	20	23	19	12
Israel	I don't enjoy working close to another.	33	22	26	23
Hungary	I don't like to work on a joint task with schoolmates.	25	22	10	19
Turkey	I don't enjoy working closely with another person.	44	22	35	27
Japan	Working closely with another person is not very satisfying.	—	12	—	3
Taiwan	Working closely with other people has never brought me pleasure.	20	13	11	11
Bangladesh	I do not find happiness in working closely with fellow workers.	19	24	19	26

ITEM 84

Country	Translation	YM	OM	YF	OF
United States	If I know that I will have to face a new situation, I will try in advance to find out as much as is possible about it.	82	84	86	86
Australia	If I know that I will have to face a new situation, I will try in advance to find out as much as is possible about it.	76	77	80	83
Germany	When I know I'm going to be facing a new situation, I try to find out as much as possible about it beforehand.	82	92	81	89
Italy	If I know that I will have to face a new situation, I will try in advance to find out as much as possible about it.	86	87	86	88
Israel	When I know that I will have to face a new situation, I try to learn as much as possible about it.	78	81	79	81
Hungary	If I know something new is about to happen, I try to prepare myself for it as well as I can.	89	84	87	89
Turkey	If I know that I will face a new situation, I try to get as much information about it as I can beforehand.	78	90	88	89
Japan	If I knew I were to enter a new situation I would thoroughly prepare for it.	—	74	—	80
Taiwan	If I know I will be facing a new situation, I will first try best to understand it.	93	88	87	94
Bangladesh	If I know that I will have to encounter a new situation then I try to find out about it in advance.	90	93	95	89

ITEM 89

Country	Translation	YM	OM	YF	OF
United States	Whenever I fail in something, I try to find out what I can do in order to avoid another failure.	85	88	87	93
Australia	Whenever I fail in something, I try to find out what I can do in order to avoid another failure.	84	83	88	85
Germany	When I fail at something, I try to find out what I can do to avoid further failure.	81	93	88	93
Italy	Anytime something goes wrong, I try to find a way so that I can do it and avoid another failure.	88	92	88	93
Israel	Each time I fail I try to find out what I could do to avoid further failure.	84	85	86	85
Hungary	If I fail at something I try to figure out what I can do to avoid another failure next time.	89	89	86	92
Turkey	When I fail in something I try to find out what I can do to avoid another failure.	80	94	91	95
Japan	When I make a mistake I plan and learn to avoid that mistake again.	—	80	—	80
Taiwan	Whenever I fail in something, I try to find out what I can do to avoid failing the next time.	87	85	80	80
Bangladesh	When I fail at something, I try to seek out the cause so that I am protected from failure the next time.	87	86	91	97

ITEM 107

Country	Translation	YM	OM	YF	OF
United States	I am certain that I will not be able to assume responsibilities for myself in the future.	19	8	12	9
Australia	I am certain that I will not be able to assume responsibilities for myself in the future.	19	16	9	11
Germany	I am certain that I will not be able to take over responsibility for myself in the future.	12	13	15	11
Italy	I am quite sure I cannot assume responsibility in the future.	16	11	13	13
Israel	I am certain that I won't be able to take care of myself in the future.	10	9	4	7
Hungary	I am sure I won't be able to take on responsibilities in the future.	10	10	5	7
Turkey	I am sure I won't be able to assume future responsibilities regarding myself.	21	13	8	14
Japan	It is certain I will assume no responsibilities for myself in the future.	—	15	—	14
Taiwan	I really believe that I will not be able to assume responsibility for myself in the future.	11	6	13	6
Bangladesh	I am certain that in the future I will not be able to acquire the capacity for being responsible even for myself.	20	13	9	19

Item 110

Country	Translation	YM	OM	YF	OF
United States	I do not rehearse how I might deal with a real coming event.	44	36	31	25
Australia	I do not rehearse how I might deal with a real coming event.	49	46	40	38
Germany	I don't worry about how I would cope with a situation that could happen to me.	28	32	43	46
Italy	I can't figure out how to tackle the situation that I am about to be confronted with.	32	19	29	18
Israel	I don't rehearse for an event that I will have to face.	42	47	51	37
Hungary	I cannot imagine how I would behave in the event of a failure situation.	30	28	28	27
Turkey	For an approaching real situation I practice (rehearse) my behavior (what I will do).	37	34	29	38
Japan	I am not going to prepare for upcoming events in my life.	—	51	—	57
Taiwan	I do not prepare for anything beforehand.	32	20	27	19
Bangladesh	I do not practice beforehand how I will contend with a realistic situation in the future.	38	34	49	35

ITEM 114

Country	Translation	YM	OM	YF	OF
United States	I do not enjoy solving difficult problems.	42	26	41	33
Australia	I do not enjoy solving difficult problems.	44	41	36	52
Germany	I don't enjoy solving hard problems.	26	18	29	23
Italy	I do not like to solve difficult problems.	42	35	47	50
Israel	I don't like solving difficult problems.	42	28	40	33
Hungary	It doesn't give me pleasure to have to solve difficult problems.	47	43	48	40
Turkey	I don't enjoy solving difficult problems.	42	34	42	53
Japan	I don't enjoy solving complex problems.	—	48	—	56
Taiwan	I don't like to solve difficult problems.	15	25	31	30
Bangladesh	I find no joy in solving complex problems.	31	23	23	20

ITEM 121

Country	Translation	YM	OM	YF	OF
United States	Worrying a little about one's future helps to make it work out better.	72	69	69	67
Australia	Worrying a little about one's future helps to make it work out better.	64	72	56	56
Germany	Worrying a little about the future helps to plan for it better.	86	89	75	78
Italy	To worry about my own future is of some help in shaping or improving my future.	85	86	81	83
Israel	Worrying a little about the future helps to plan for it better.	79	81	71	70
Hungary	If the future makes me uneasy, it just makes me work all the harder to make it better.	78	77	81	79
Turkey	It helps a person to be concerned about his/her future.	69	89	78	79
Japan	To worry a little about the future will help to make it work better.	—	96	—	95
Taiwan	Planning for the future will enhance one's future accomplishments.	93	89	82	92
Bangladesh	A certain amount of anxiety about the future is helpful toward conducting one's life well.	81	92	92	95

Individual Values
(They do not constitute a scale.)

---

5. I would not hurt someone just for the "heck of it."

40. I blame others even when I know that I am at fault too. (−)

48. Telling the truth means nothing to me. (−)

67. I do not care how my actions affect others as long as I gain something. (−)

83. I like to help a friend whenever I can.

120. I would not like to be associated with those kids who "hit below the belt."

ITEM 5

Country	Translation	YM	OM	YF	OF
United States	I would not hurt someone just for the "heck of it."	66	83	90	86
Australia	I would not hurt someone just for the "heck of it."	63	78	72	81
Germany	I would not injure anyone just simply for the fun of it.	65	64	63	75
Italy	I would never hurt anybody for the mere pleasure of doing so.	68	79	78	86
Israel	I would not hurt somebody just for the fun of it.	59	73	75	82
Hungary	I would not like to hurt anyone just for fun.	58	61	68	69
Turkey	I would not offend anyone by saying "I don't care."	82	90	87	83
Japan	I will not harm an individual because of my own frustrations.	—	68	—	64
Taiwan	I will not hurt someone as a result of my anger.	72	62	60	69
Bangladesh	I never strike someone only to hurt them.	62	58	69	65

ITEM 40

Country	Translation	YM	OM	YF	OF
United States	I blame others even when I know that I am at fault too.	35	24	31	26
Australia	I blame others even when I know that I am at fault too.	45	29	36	30
Germany	I accuse others even when I know that I am the one at fault.	19	11	14	9
Italy	I criticize other people when I know I am guilty, too.	44	37	41	29
Israel	I blame others, even when I know that I too am guilty.	29	25	17	15
Hungary	I blame others even if I am also at fault.	16	17	5	7
Turkey	Even if I know that I am also guilty, I will put the blame on (someone else) others.	13	11	12	7
Japan	Even if I know I'm guilty, I'll blame someone else.	—	15	—	19
Taiwan	Even if I know I'm wrong, I still blame others.	24	25	31	27
Bangladesh	Even if I know that I am to blame, I do not desist from blaming others.	31	29	18	20

ITEM 48

Country	Translation	YM	OM	YF	OF
United States	Telling the truth means nothing to me.	13	7	12	7
Australia	Telling the truth means nothing to me.	28	19	19	13
Germany	It is not important for me to tell the truth.	30	18	20	12
Italy	To say truth makes no sense.	24	16	18	14
Israel	For me there is no value in telling the truth.	21	14	8	11
Hungary	Truthfulness doesn't mean anything to me.	13	14	9	7
Turkey	Telling the truth doesn't mean anything to me.	7	9	6	2
Japan	Telling the truth is not an important matter to me.	—	12	—	9
Taiwan	Telling the truth has little meaning to me.	15	14	20	16
Bangladesh	It seems to me unprofitable to speak the truth at all times.	15	21	31	24

ITEM 67

Country	Translation	YM	OM	YF	OF
United States	I do not care how my actions affect others as long as I gain something.	20	11	7	6
Australia	I do not care how my actions affect others as long as I gain something.	32	22	17	11
Germany	I don't care how my actions affect others as long as I can have an advantage.	22	7	11	8
Italy	I don't worry about what my actions are doing to others providing I derive some benefit.	13	10	9	7
Israel	I don't care how my acts affect others as long as I profit.	39	31	20	18
Hungary	I do not care how my actions affect others, as long as I benefit from them.	16	25	9	12
Turkey	I don't care how my actions affect others as long as I gain something from it.	32	33	24	30
Japan	If I can gain something, I would not care how my actions affect others.	—	19	—	20
Taiwan	If I can get something, I don't mind how my actions will affect others.	13	13	9	14
Bangladesh	I don't care about loss of others for my own gain.	36	23	17	10

ITEM 83

Country	Translation	YM	OM	YF	OF
United States	I like to help a friend whenever I can.	90	93	97	96
Australia	I like to help a friend whenever I can.	93	93	92	96
Germany	I am glad to help a friend whenever I can.	87	89	95	92
Italy	I like to help a friend when I can.	86	90	93	95
Israel	When I can, I like to help a friend.	90	94	92	95
Hungary	I always like to help my friends.	87	88	95	95
Turkey	I enjoy helping my friends as much as I can.	89	95	94	100
Japan	I would like to help my friends as much as possible.	—	86	—	93
Taiwan	I am willing to do all I can to help my friends.	98	91	93	93
Bangladesh	I like helping friends whenever I can.	89	90	96	92

ITEM 120

Country	Translation	YM	OM	YF	OF
United States	I would not like to be associated with those kids who "hit below the belt."	71	71	69	74
Australia	I would not like to be associated with those kids who "hit below the belt."	62	75	60	54
Germany	I wouldn't like to hang around young people who "hit below the belt." (who are unfair and mean).	80	75	77	77
Italy	I would not like to be compared to kids that cheat in competition.	69	75	74	78
Israel	I would not like to be considered as someone who doesn't play fair.	76	78	68	71
Hungary	I wouldn't like to belong to a group that "hits below the belt."	80	80	79	86
Turkey	I do not enjoy being with other children who are "lowly bastards."	74	82	71	85
Japan	I don't like to be associated with unfair people.	—	82	—	79
Taiwan	I will not associate with those who are not straight.	82	90	89	90
Bangladesh	I do not like being with boys and girls who break the rules.	69	85	84	88

Table of Alphas

Psychological Self (PS-1)
ALPHA: IMPULSE CONTROL

Sample	Younger males	Older males	Younger females	Older females
U.S.	61	68	66	60
Australia	25	51	63	52
Germany	53	52	55	62
Italy	57	62	54	60
Israel	43	73	53	70
Hungary	53	53	62	69
Turkey	03	62	56	60
Japan	—	56	—	72
Taiwan	40	54	28	53
Bangladesh	54	48	34	50

Psychological Self (PS-2)
ALPHA: EMOTIONAL TONE

Sample	Younger males	Older males	Younger females	Older females
U.S.	72	71	79	81
Australia	62	71	77	75
Germany	72	74	77	74
Italy	69	68	76	76
Israel	73	81	76	82
Hungary	74	79	77	81
Turkey	70	75	80	77
Japan	—	67	—	71
Taiwan	50	76	61	83
Bangladesh	56	61	58	65

Psychological Self (PS-3)
ALPHA: BODY AND SELF-IMAGE

Sample	Younger males	Older males	Younger females	Older females
U.S.	64	63	72	75
Australia	50	66	66	63
Germany	53	65	49	60
Italy	54	58	53	62
Israel	53	73	67	65
Hungary	54	56	60	59
Turkey	37	55	62	60
Japan	—	64	—	42
Taiwan	65	51	30	52
Bangladesh	39	52	41	52

Social Self (SS-1)
ALPHA: SOCIAL RELATIONSHIPS

Sample	Younger males	Older males	Younger females	Older females
U.S.	69	74	67	71
Australia	48	65	61	72
Germany	65	72	65	65
Italy	62	65	62	72
Israel	70	79	69	74
Hungary	72	73	69	73
Turkey	55	60	64	63
Japan	—	72	—	77
Taiwan	48	70	67	63
Bangladesh	51	56	58	61

Social Self (SS-2)
ALPHA: VOCATIONAL–EDUCATIONAL GOALS

Sample	Younger males	Older males	Younger females	Older females
U.S.	70	63	69	70
Australia	49	52	51	57
Germany	59	66	46	61
Italy	51	55	58	52
Israel	31	54	62	32
Hungary	65	59	53	58
Turkey	41	50	63	58
Japan	—	63	—	64
Taiwan	60	66	38	59
Bangladesh	46	45	41	55

Sexual Self (S×S)
ALPHA: SEXUAL ATTITUDES

Sample	Younger males	Older males	Younger females	Older females
U.S.	65	54	66	67
Australia	61	61	65	62
Germany	48	58	55	68
Italy	71	64	59	67
Israel	71	65	62	59
Hungary	70	67	73	69
Turkey	73	64	60	53
Japan	—	69	—	72
Taiwan	48	52	49	54
Bangladesh	44	64	61	59

Familial Self (FS)
ALPHA: FAMILY RELATIONSHIPS

Sample	Younger males	Older males	Younger females	Older females
U.S.	84	81	88	89
Australia	80	81	84	88
Germany	79	84	77	85
Italy	79	72	85	84
Israel	81	83	86	85
Hungary	83	83	82	85
Turkey	70	73	81	80
Japan	—	79	—	84
Taiwan	82	82	86	80
Bangladesh	62	71	79	74

Coping Self (CS-1)
ALPHA: MASTERY OF THE EXTERNAL WORLD

Sample	Younger males	Older males	Younger females	Older females
U.S.	58	55	55	61
Australia	48	37	37	47
Germany	36	49	41	51
Italy	42	49	48	56
Israel	46	62	45	43
Hungary	59	57	48	60
Turkey	39	53	52	39
Japan	—	62	—	57
Taiwan	27	60	10	54
Bangladesh	28	47	46	44

Coping Self (CS-2)
ALPHA: PSYCHOPATHOLOGY

Sample	Younger males	Older males	Younger females	Older females
U.S.	71	68	71	71
Australia	53	63	60	68
Germany	56	65	62	59
Italy	54	42	47	41
Israel	65	70	63	70
Hungary	58	56	60	64
Turkey	55	65	67	64
Japan	—	54	—	68
Taiwan	69	61	63	68
Bangladesh	63	56	46	58

Coping Self (CS-3)
ALPHA: SUPERIOR ADJUSTMENT

Sample	Younger males	Older males	Younger females	Older females
U.S.	60	59	65	62
Australia	45	53	51	59
Germany	36	55	29	50
Italy	60	63	69	69
Israel	60	50	49	50
Hungary	48	56	53	51
Turkey	47	58	44	41
Japan	—	49	—	55
Taiwan	77	77	71	74
Bangladesh	54	62	52	57

Means Table

The raw scores of the different scales for the ten countries studied are presented in this section. The scores were all reversed so that in these tables, the higher the score, the better the self-image.

Sample	Younger males	Older males	Younger females	Older females
Australia	3.96	4.26	3.75	3.91
Bangladesh	3.94	3.93	3.63	3.79
Hungary	4.57	4.44	4.36	4.11
Israel	4.37	4.46	4.12	4.06
Italy	3.77	4.01	3.54	3.72
Japan	—	3.83	—	3.74
Taiwan	3.98	4.08	3.66	3.86
Turkey	4.39	4.52	3.99	3.96
United States	4.30	4.51	4.13	4.22
West Germany	4.56	4.45	4.14	4.12

EMOTIONAL TONE

Sample	Younger males	Older males	Younger females	Older females
Australia	4.35	4.29	4.12	4.12
Bangladesh	3.91	3.92	3.65	3.47
Hungary	4.81	4.52	4.69	4.35
Israel	4.66	4.49	4.33	4.23
Italy	4.37	4.33	4.06	4.02
Japan	—	3.64	—	3.58
Taiwan	4.17	4.09	4.08	3.90
Turkey	4.32	4.30	4.16	4.02
United States	4.47	4.50	4.36	4.37
West Germany	4.80	4.45	4.41	4.34

BODY IMAGE

Sample	Younger males	Older males	Younger females	Older females
Australia	4.29	4.29	3.92	3.94
Bangladesh	3.88	3.68	3.79	3.58
Hungary	4.20	4.22	4.19	4.01
Israel	4.51	4.47	4.49	4.39
Italy	4.50	4.48	4.10	4.22
Japan	—	3.77	—	3.61
Taiwan	3.89	4.06	3.85	3.98
Turkey	4.34	4.43	4.20	4.20
United States	4.51	4.55	4.35	4.41
West Germany	4.63	4.54	4.29	4.42

SOCIAL RELATIONSHIPS

Sample	Younger males	Older males	Younger females	Older females
Australia	4.59	4.56	4.57	4.59
Bangladesh	4.34	4.34	4.33	4.36
Hungary	4.85	4.64	4.93	4.61
Israel	4.48	4.48	4.61	4.58
Italy	4.50	4.44	4.32	4.38
Japan	—	3.96	—	4.06
Taiwan	4.20	4.15	4.14	4.10
Turkey	4.17	4.39	4.40	4.45
United States	4.51	4.74	4.68	4.67
West Germany	4.64	4.39	4.56	4.68

SEXUAL ATTITUDES

Sample	Younger males	Older males	Younger females	Older females
Australia	4.65	4.60	3.91	4.08
Bangladesh	3.48	3.83	3.25	3.50
Hungary	4.29	4.55	3.73	4.07
Israel	4.56	4.42	4.16	4.12
Italy	4.69	4.66	3.82	4.11
Japan	—	3.94	—	3.51
Taiwan	3.51	4.03	3.08	3.19
Turkey	3.85	4.29	3.20	3.55
United States	4.44	4.53	4.01	4.19
West Germany	4.30	4.32	3.98	4.17

FAMILY RELATIONSHIPS

Sample	Younger males	Older males	Younger females	Older females
Australia	4.47	4.56	4.37	4.30
Bangladesh	4.63	4.70	4.75	4.65
Hungary	4.81	4.51	4.92	4.71
Israel	4.76	4.76	4.81	4.79
Italy	4.81	4.75	4.60	4.62
Japan	—	4.23	—	4.15
Taiwan	4.55	4.65	4.50	4.55
Turkey	4.77	4.85	4.69	4.81
United States	4.66	4.74	4.63	4.63
West Germany	4.69	4.53	4.46	4.52

MASTERY OF THE EXTERNAL WORLD

Sample	Younger males	Older males	Younger females	Older females
Australia	4.61	4.56	4.41	4.50
Bangladesh	4.52	4.60	4.59	4.46
Hungary	4.87	4.73	4.79	4.65
Israel	4.96	4.79	4.89	4.87
Italy	4.64	4.69	4.54	4.60
Japan	—	3.87	—	3.79
Taiwan	4.44	4.28	4.15	4.18
Turkey	4.60	4.86	4.52	4.63
United States	4.86	4.98	4.91	4.91
West Germany	4.69	4.76	4.45	4.65

VOCATIONAL AND EDUCATIONAL GOALS

Sample	Younger males	Older males	Younger females	Older females
Australia	4.80	4.79	4.92	4.95
Bangladesh	4.86	4.84	4.94	4.85
Hungary	4.69	4.43	4.84	4.67
Israel	4.63	4.66	4.82	4.82
Italy	4.93	4.82	4.99	4.97
Japan	—	4.57	—	4.69
Taiwan	4.72	4.81	4.90	4.93
Turkey	4.79	4.88	4.97	5.03
United States	4.81	5.03	5.08	5.12
West Germany	4.80	4.81	4.75	4.79

PSYCHOPATHOLOGY

Sample	Younger males	Older males	Younger females	Older females
Australia	4.36	4.50	4.20	4.18
Bangladesh	4.11	4.13	3.97	3.92
Hungary	4.80	4.71	4.76	4.56
Israel	4.71	4.67	4.65	4.53
Italy	4.56	4.65	4.19	4.29
Japan	—	4.11	—	4.00
Taiwan	4.18	4.15	4.05	3.95
Turkey	4.14	4.42	4.14	4.27
United States	4.55	4.64	4.48	4.55
West Germany	4.69	4.79	4.52	4.78

SUPERIOR ADJUSTMENT

Sample	Younger males	Older males	Younger females	Older females
Australia	4.26	4.32	4.43	4.38
Bangladesh	4.50	4.75	4.72	4.73
Hungary	4.46	4.33	4.62	4.51
Israel	4.40	4.45	4.47	4.45
Italy	4.43	4.50	4.37	4.47
Japan	—	4.06	—	4.14
Taiwan	4.52	4.60	4.59	4.62
Turkey	4.28	4.58	4.51	4.48
United States	4.41	4.57	4.57	4.64
West Germany	4.48	4.52	4.32	4.52

APPENDIX 4

Depression Scale

A depression scale was constructed for the purpose of studying one major psychopathological state. Alphas for this scale are shown in the following pages.

Item No.	English version of the item[a]
45.	I feel empty emotionally most of the time.
61.	I often feel that I would rather die than go on living.
66.	I feel so very lonely.
103.	I find life an endless series of problems—without solution in sight.
130.	I frequently feel sad.

[a]Back-translations of the items can be seen in Appendix 1.

ALPHAS FOR DEPRESSION

Country	Younger males	Older males	Younger females	Older females
United States	0.76	0.77	0.81	0.80
Australia	0.68	0.61	0.73	0.83
Germany	0.65	0.77	0.61	0.68
Italy	0.64	0.66	0.74	0.73
Israel	0.64	0.73	0.76	0.74
Hungary	0.67	0.69	0.73	0.69
Turkey	0.63	0.79	0.72	0.77
Japan	—	0.69	—	0.77
Taiwan	0.72	0.75	0.81	0.84
Bangladesh	0.64	0.56	0.67	0.67

PERCENT ENDORSEMENT FOR THE FIVE ITEMS CONSTITUTING
THE DEPRESSION SCALE[a]

Country	Younger males	Older males	Younger females	Older females	Mean
United States	16	18	25	20	20
Australia	27	23	35	34	30
Germany	17	11	17	11	14
Italy	15	18	34	23	22
Israel	17	19	18	29	21
Hungary	10	18	12	19	15
Turkey	33	37	33	42	36
Japan	—	45	—	44	22
Taiwan	23	38	27	38	31
Bangladesh	42	42	52	56	48
Average	22	27	28	32	27

[a]Percentages have been rounded to the nearest whole number.

References

N. Albert and A. T. Beck, Incidence of Depression in Early Adolescence: A Preliminary Study, *Journal of Youth and Adolescence*, 4 (1975), 301–107.

P. Aries, *Centuries of Childhood* (New York: Vintage Books, 1962).

A. Bandura, *Social Learning Theory* (Englewood Cliffs, NJ: Prentice-Hall, 1977).

R. Benedict, *Patterns of Culture* (Boston: Houghton Mifflin, 1934).

P. Berger and T. Luckmann, *The Social Construction of Reality* (New York: Doubleday, 1966).

J. W. Berry, Introduction to Methodology, *Handbook of Cross-Cultural Psychology: 2. Methodology*, H. C. Triandis and J. W. Berry (Eds.) (Boston: Allyn & Bacon, 1980).

S. Bjornsson, Epidemiological Investigation of Mental Disorders of Children in Reykjavik, Iceland, *Scandinavian Journal of Psychology*, 15 (1974), 244–254.

J. Block, *Lives through Time* (Berkeley: Bancroft Books, 1971).

P. Blos, *On Adolescence* (New York: Free Press of Glencoe, 1961).

J. H. Boyd and M. M. Weissman, Epidemiology of Affective Disorders: A Reexamination and Future Directions, *Archives of General Psychiatry*, 38 (1981), 1039–1046.

M. H. Brenner, Mortality and the National Economy: A Review and the Experience of England and Wales, 1936–1976, *Lancet*, 2 (1979), 568–573.

R. Brislin, Translation and Content Analysis of Oral and Written Materials, *Handbook of Cross-Cultural Psychology: 2. Methodology*, H. C. Triandis and J. W. Berry (Eds.) (Boston: Allyn & Bacon, 1980).

R. Brislin, Cross-Cultural Research in psychology, *Annual Review of Psychology*, 34 (1983), 363–400.

J. Casagrande, The Ends of Translation, *International Journal of American Linguistics*, 20 (1954), 335–340.

N. Chomsky, *Syntactic Structures* (The Hague: Mouton, 1957).

N. Chomsky, *Reflections on Language* (New York: Pantheon, 1975).

N. Chomsky, *Rules and Regulations* (New York: Columbia University Press, 1980).

E. Clifford, Body Satisfaction in Adolescence, *Perceptual and Motor Skills*, 33 (1971), 119–125.

F. E. Crumley, The Adolescent Suicide Attempt: A Cardinal Symptom of a Serious Psychiatric Disorder, *American Journal of Psychotherapy*, 36 (1982), 158–165.

R. G. D'Andrade, Cultural Meaning Systems, *Culture Theory: Essays on Mind, Self, and Emotion*, R. A. Shweder and R. A. Levine (Eds.) (Cambridge: Cambridge University Press, 1984).

A. Davidson, J. J. Jaccard, H. C. Triandis, M. L. Morales, and R. Diaz-Guerrero, Cross-Cultural Model Testing: Toward a Solution of the Etic-Emic Dilemma, *International Journal of Psychology*, 11 (1976), 1–13.

Diagnostic and Statistical Manual of Mental Disorders, 3rd ed. (Washington: American Psychiatric Association, 1980).

J. A. Doane, K. L. West, M. J. Goldstein, E. H. Rodnick, and J. E. Jones, Parental Communication Deviance and Affective Style: Predictors of Subsequent Schizophrenia

Spectrum Disorders in Vulnerable Adolescents, *AMA Archives of General Psychiatry, 38* (1981), 679–685.

L. T. Doi, The Japanese Patterns of Communication and the Concept of Amae, *Quarterly Journal of Speech, 59* (1973), 180–185.

E. Douvan and J. Adelson, *The Adolescent Experience* (New York: John Wiley and Sons, 1966).

R. A. Easterlin, *Birth and Fortune* (New York: Basic Books, 1980).

M. Eliade, *Myth and Reality* (New York: Harper & Row, 1963).

E. H. Erikson, *Childhood and Society* (New York: W. W. Norton, 1950).

E. Erikson, *Insight and Responsibility* (New York: W. W. Norton, 1964).

E. Erikson, *Toys and Reasons: Stages in the Ritualization of Experience* (New York: W. W. Norton, 1977).

E. Erikson, *The Life Cycle Completed* (New York: W. W. Norton, 1982).

B. N. Ezeiloi, Cross-Cultural Utility of the Tennessee Self-Concept Scale, *Psychological Reports, 51*(3) (1982), 897–898.

N. L. Farberow, Adolescent Suicide, *The Adolescent Mood Disturbances*, H. Golombek (Ed.) (New York: International Universities Press, 1983).

M. Forbes, Editorial, *Forbes* magazine (December 1, 1951).

J. N. Franco, A Developmental Analysis of Self-Concept in Mexican American and Anglo School Children, *Hispanic Journal of Behavioral Sciences, 5*(2) (1983), 207–218.

D. X. Freedman, Psychiatric Epidemiology Count, *Archives of General Psychiatry, 41* (1984), 931–933.

A. Freud, Adolescence, *Psychoanalytic Study of the Child, 13* (1958), 255–278.

S. Freud, *An Outline of Psychoanalysis* (New York: W. W. Norton, 1949).

P. S. Fry, The Development of Differentiation in Self-Evaluations: A Cross-Cultural Study, *Journal of Psychology, 87*(2) (1974), 193–202.

A. Furnham and R. Karris, Self-image, Disparity, Ethnic Identity and Sex-Role Stereotypes in British and Cypriot Adolescents, *Journal of Adolescence 6*(3) (1983), 275–292.

H. Gardner, *Frames of Mind: The Theory of Multiple Intelligences* (New York: Basic Books, 1985).

C. Geertz, *The Interpretation of Cultures* (New York: Basic Books, 1973).

C. Geertz, From the Native's Point of View: On the Nature of Anthropological Understanding, *Culture Theory*, R. A. Shweder and R. A. LeVine (Eds.) (New York: Cambridge University Press, 1984).

C. Gilligan, *In a Different Voice* (Cambridge: Harvard University Press, 1982).

E. Goffman, *The Presentation of Self in Everyday Life* (New York: Doubleday, 1959).

P. Graham and M. Rutter, Psychiatric Disorder in the Young Adolescent: A Follow-Up Study, *Proceedings of the Royal Society of Medicine, 66* (1973), 58–61.

G. Granzberg, Television and Self-Concept Formation in Developing Areas: The Central Canadian Algonkian Experience, *Journal of Cross-Cultural Psychology, 16*(3) (1985), 313–328.

R. D. Gregory, Self-Concept across Sex, Color, and Teacher-Estimated, Annual Family Income Level for Students in Grades Seven through Twelve, *Dissertation Abstracts International, 38* (1977), 1859.

G. S. Hall, *Adolescence: Its Psychology and Its Relation to Physiology, Anthropology, Sociology, Sex, Crime, Religion and Education* (New York: D. Appleton, 1904).

I. D. Harris and K. I. Howard, Correlates of Perceived Parental Favoritism, *Journal of Psychology, 146* (1985), 45–56.

M. Harris, *Cows, Pigs, Wars and Witches: The Riddles of Culture* (New York: Random House, 1974).

S. Hartlage, K. I. Howard, and E. Ostrov, The Mental Health Professional and the Normal Adolescent, *Patterns of Adolescent Self-Image*, D. Offer, E. Ostrov, and K. I. Howard (Eds.) (San Francisco: Jossey-Bass, 1984).

G. W. Healey and R. R. Deblassie, A Comparison of Negro, Anglo, and Spanish-American Adolescents' Self-Concept, *Adolescence 9* (1974), 15–24.

D. J. Helland, Sex-Role Correlates of Adolescent Self-Esteem, *Dissertation Abstracts International, 34* (1973), 2026–2027.

H. Hendin, *Suicide in America* (New York: W. W. Norton, 1982).

B. Hille, Possibilities for Social Science Comparisons between the Two Generations, *Psychologische Randschau, 32*(3) (1981), 180–199.

P. C. Holinger and D. Offer, Prediction of Adolescent Suicide: A Population Model, *American Journal of Psychiatry, 139*(3) (March 1982), 302–307.

P. C. Holinger, D. Offer, and E. Ostrov, Suicide and Homicide in the United States: An Epidemiological Study of Violent Death, Population Change, and the Potential for Prediction, *American Journal of Psychiatry, 144*(2) (February 1987), 215–219.

P. C. Holinger, D. Offer, and M. A. Zola, A Prediction Model of Suicide Among Youth, *Journal of Nervous and Mental Disease, 8,* 1987.

R. W. Hudgens, *Psychiatric Disorders in Adolescents* (Baltimore: Williams and Wilkins, 1974).

Institute of Medicine, Discussion Summary from Workshop on Forecasting Stress-Related Social Problems, *National Academy of Sciences, Division of Mental Health and Behavioral Medicine,* (Washington, D.C., September 26–27, 1985).

S. Irvine and W. K. Carroll, Testing and Assessment across Cultures: Issues in Methodology and Theory, *Handbook of Cross-Cultural Psychology: 2. Methodology,* H. C. Triandis and J. W. Berry (Eds.) (Boston: Allyn & Bacon, 1980).

W. James, *The Principles of Psychology* (Cambridge: Harvard University Press, 1890) (1983).

C. G. Jung, *The Stages of Life: Modern Man in Search of a Soul* (New York: Harcourt, Brace, & World, 1933).

C. G. Jung, *The Archetypes and the Collective Unconscious* (Princeton: Princeton University Press, 1959).

C. G. Jung, *Memories, Dreams, Reflections* (New York: Random House, 1961).

D. B. Kandel and M. Davies, Epidemiology of Depressive Mood in Adolescents, *Archives of General Psychiatry, 39* (1982), 1205–1212.

G. A. Kelly, *The Psychology of Personal Constructs* (New York: W. W. Norton, 1955).

M. Kertész, D. Offer, E. Ostrov, and K. I. Howard, Hungarian Adolescents' Self-Concepts, *Journal of Youth and Adolescence, 15*(3) (1986), 275–286.

L. Kohlberg, *The Philosophy of Moral Development* (San Francisco: Harper & Row, 1981).

L. Kohlberg and C. Gilligan, The Adolescent as Philosopher: The Discovery of the Self in a Post-Conventional World, *Daedalus, 100* (1971), 1051–1086.

H. Kohut, *Self Psychology and the Humanities* (New York: W. W. Norton, 1985).

J. Krupinski, A. G. Baikie, A. Stoller, J. Graves, D. M. O'Day, and P. Polke, A Community Health Survey of Heyfield, Victoria, *Medical Journal of Australia, 54* (1967), 1204–1211.

G. T. Kurian, *The New Book of World Ranking* (New York: Facts on File Publications, 1984).

W. W. Lambert, Introduction to Perspectives, *Handbook of Cross-Cultural Psychology: 1. Perspectives* (Boston: Allyn & Bacon, 1980).

T. S. Langner, J. C. Gersten, and J. G. Eisenberg, Approaches to Measurement and Definition in Epidemiology of Behavior Disorders: Ethnic Background and Child Behavior, *International Journal of Health Services, 4* (1974), 483–501.

D. Lee, Notes on the Conception of the Self Among the Wintu Indians, *Journal of Abnormal and Social Psychology, 45* (1950), 538–543.

R. LeVine, *Culture, Behavior, Personality* (New York: Aldine, 1982).

C. Levi-Strauss, *The Savage Mind* (Chicago: University of Chicago Press, 1966).

R. J. Lifton, A Nuclear Age Ethos: The Psychological-Ethical Principles, *Journal of Humanistic Psychology, 25* (1985), 39–40.

A. Locksley and E. Douvan, Problem Behavior in Adolescents, *Gender and Disordered Behavior,* E. Gombera and V. Frank (Eds.) (New York: Brunner/Mazel, 1979).

W. J. Lonner, The Search for Psychological Universals, *Handbook of Cross-Cultural Psychology: 1. Perspectives,* H. C. Triandis and J. W. Berry (Eds.) (Boston: Allyn & Bacon, 1980).

W. J. Lonner, Television in the Developing World Introduction, *Journal of Cross-Cultural Psychology, 16*(3) (1985), 259–262.

P. A. Marks and D. L. Haller, Now I Lay Me Down for Keeps: A Study of Adolescent Suicide Attempts, *Journal of Clinical Psychology, 33* (1977), 390–400.

E. Marshall, Nuclear Winter Debate Heats Up, *Science,* (January 16, 1987), 271–273.

J. F. Masterson, *The Psychiatric Dilemma of Adolescence* (Boston: Little, Brown, 1967).

G. H. Mead, *Mind, Self and Society* (Chicago: University of Chicago Press, 1934).

M. McLuhan and Q. Fiore, *The Medium Is the Message* (New York: Bantam Books, 1967).

M. Mead, *Coming of Age in Samoa* (New York: William Morrow, 1928).

M. Mead, *Culture and Commitment* (New York: Doubleday, 1978).

G. D. Mellinger, M. B. Balter, D. I. Manheimer, et al., Psychic Distress, Life Crisis, and Use of Psychotherapeutic Medications: National Household Survey Data, *Archives of General Psychiatry, 35* (1978), 1045–1052.

J. K. Meyers, M. M. Weissman, G. L. Tischler, C. E. Holzer, III, P. J. Leaf, H. Orvaschel, J. C. Anthony, J. H. Boyd, J. D. Burke, Jr., M. Kramer, and R. Stoltzman, Six-Month Prevalence of Psychiatric Disorders in Three Communities, *Archives of General Psychiatry, 41* (1984), 959–978.

W. Mischel, Self-Control and the Self, *The Self: Psychological and Philosophical Issues,* T. Mischel (Ed.) (Totowa, NJ: Rowman and Littlefield, 1977).

J. R. Mitchell, Normality in Adolescence, *Adolescent Psychiatry, 8* (1980), 201–213.

R. H. Monge, Developmental Trends in Factors of Adolescent Self-Concept, *Developmental Psychology, 8* (1973), 382–393.

R. L. Monroe and R. H. Monroe, Population Density and Affective Relationships in Three East African Societies, *Journal of Social Psychology, 88* (1972), 15–20.

K. E. Musa and M. E. Roach, Adolescent Appearance and Self-Concept, *Adolescence, 8* (1973), 385–394.

A. Newell, Duncker on Thinking: An Inquiry into Progress in Cognition, *A Century of Psychology as Science,* S. Koch and D. E. Leary (Eds.) (New York: McGraw-Hill, 1985).

B. J. Newton and E. B. Buck, Television as Significant Other: Its Relationship to Self-Descriptors in Five Countries, *Journal of Cross-Cultural Psychology, 16*(3) (1985), 289–312.

D. Offer, *The Psychological World of the Teenager: A Study of Normal Adolescent Boys* (New York: Basic Books, 1969).

D. Offer and J. B. Offer, *From Teenage to Young Manhood: A Psychological Study* (New York: Basic Books, 1975).

D. Offer, E. Ostrov, and K. I. Howard, *The Adolescent: A Psychological Self-Portrait* (New York: Basic Books, 1981a).

D. Offer, E. Ostrov, and K. I. Howard, The Mental Health Professional's Concept of the Normal Adolescent, *Archives of General Psychiatry, 38* (1981b), 149–152.

D. Offer, E. Ostrov, and K. I. Howard, *The Offer Self-Image for Adolescents: A Manual*, Special Publication (Chicago: Michael Reese Hospital and Medical Center, 1982).

D. Offer, E. Ostrov, and K. I. Howard, *Patterns of Adolescent Self-Image* (San Francisco: Jossey-Bass, 1984).

D. Offer, E. Ostrov, and K. I. Howard, Normal Adolescents' Concern with Nuclear Issues, Unpublished manuscript (Chicago: Michael Reese Hospital and Medical Center, 1986a).

D. Offer, E. Ostrov, and K. I. Howard, Self-Image, Delinquency and Help Seeking Behavior Among Normal Adolescents, *Adolescent Psychiatry, 13*, S. Feinstein (Ed.) (Chicago: University of Chicago Press, 1986b).

D. Offer, E. Ostrov, and K. I. Howard, The Epidemiology of Mental Health and Mental Illness among Urban Adolescents, *Significant Advances in Child Psychiatry*, J. Call (Ed.) (in press, 1987).

D. Offer and R. P. Spiro, The Disturbed Adolescent Goes to College, *Journal of American College Health Association, 35* (1987), 209–214.

A. A. Olowu, A Cross-Cultural Study of Adolescent Self-Concept, *Journal of Adolescence, 6(3)* (1983), 263–274.

E. Ostrov, Loneliness, Shyness, and Withdrawal in Adolescence, *Advances in Adolescent Mental Health, 1* (B) *Mental Health Disorders in Adolescence*, R. Feldman and A. Stiffman (Eds.) (1986).

Oxford English Dictionary (Oxford: Clarendon Press, 1983).

U. Parek and T. V. Rao, Cross-Cultural Surveys and Interviewing, *Handbook of Cross-Cultural Psychology: 2. Methodology*, H. C. Triandis and J. W. Berry (Eds.) (Boston: Allyn & Bacon, 1980).

M. L. Peck, The Loner: An Exploration of a Suicidal Subtype in Adolescence, *Adolescent Psychiatry, 9* (1981), 461–466.

M. Peck, Youth Suicide, *Death Education, 6* (1982), 29–47.

J. Piaget, *Six Psychological Studies* (New York: Vintage Books, 1967).

J. Piaget, *Structuralism* (New York: Harper & Row, 1970).

J. Piaget, Need and Significance of Cross-Cultural Studies in Genetic Psychology, *Culture and Cognition Readings in Cross-Cultural Psychology*, J. Berry and P. Dasen (Eds.) (London: Methuen, 1973).

K. Pike, *Language in Relation to a Unified Theory of the Structure of Human Behavior* (The Hague: Mouton, 1966).

H. G. Rabichow and M. A. Sklansky, *Effective Counseling of Adolescents* (Chicago: Follett, 1980).

T. H. Rodriguez, J. Behar, C. Martinez, and F. Barioud, Dimension of Personal Identity in Adolescence: A Comparative Study, *Revista de Psicologia General y Aplicads, 37(3)* (1982), 507–527.

C. Rogers, *A Way of Being* (Boston: Houghton Mifflin, 1980).

M. Rutter, *Changing Youth in a Changing Society* (Cambridge: Harvard University Press, 1980).

M. Rutter, P. Graham, D. F. D. Chadwick, and W. Yule, Adolescent Turmoil: Fact or Fiction, *Journal of Child Psychology and Psychiatry, 17* (1976), 35–56.

A. Schrut, Suicidal Adolescents and Children, *Journal of the American Medical Association, 188* (1964), 1103–1107.

R. Sennett (Ed.), *The Psychology of Society* (New York: Vintage Books, 1977).

C. B. Smith, A. J. Weigart, and D. L. Thomas, Self-Esteem and Religiosity: An Analysis of Catholic Adolescents from Five Cultures, *Journal for the Scientific Study of Religion, 18(1)* (1979), 51–60.

M. E. Spiro, Some Reflections on Cultural Determinism and Relativism with Special

Reference to Emotion and Reason, *Culture Theory: Essays on Mind, Self, and Emotion*, R. A. Sweder and R. A. LeVine (Eds.) (New York: Cambridge University Press, 1984).

N. Tabachnick, The Interlocking Psychologies of Suicide and Adolescence, *Adolescent Psychiatry*, 9 (1981), 399–410.

H. C. Triandis, *The Analysis of Subjective Culture* (New York: John Wiley, 1972).

H. C. Triandis, Some Universals of Social Behavior, *Personality and Social Psychology Bulletin*, 4 (1978), 1–16.

H. C. Triandis, The Future of Cross-Cultural Psychology, *Perspectives in Cross-Cultural Psychology*, A. J. Marsella, R. C. Thorp, and T. J. Ciborowski (Eds.) (New York: Academic Press, 1979).

H. C. Triandis, Introduction to Handbook of Cross-Cultural Psychology, *Handbook of Cross-Cultural Psychology*, 1, H. C. Triandis and J. W. Berry (Eds.) (Boston: Allyn & Bacon, 1980).

H. C. Triandis and R. W. Brislin, Cross-Cultural Psychology, *American Psychologist*, 39(9) (1984), 1006–1016.

C. Turnbull, *The Human Cycle* (New York: Simon & Schuster, 1983).

UNESCO, *Statistical Yearbook* (New York: United Nations, UNESCO, 1984).

United Nations, *Statistical Indicators on Youth* (New York: United Nations, 1985).

G. E. Vaillant, *Adaptation to Life* (Boston: Little, Brown, 1977).

G. E. Vaillant and C. C. McArthur, Natural History of Male Psychological Health: 1. The Adult Life Cycle from 18–50, *Seminars in Psychiatry*, 4 (1972), 4–16.

I. B. Weiner and A. C. DelGaudio, Psychopathology in Adolescence, *Archives of General Psychiatry*, 33 (1976), 187–193.

W. A. Westley and N. B. Epstein, *The Silent Majority* (San Francisco: Jossey Bass, 1969).

J. Whiting, Methods and Problems in Cross-Cultural Research, *Handbook of Social Psychology*, 2, G. Lindzey and E. Aronson (Eds.) (Reading, MA: Addison-Wesley, 1968).

R. G. Wiggins, Differences in Self-Perceptions in Ninth-Grade Boys and Girls, *Adolescence*, 8 (1973), 491–496.

T. Williams, Implications of a Natural Experiment in the Developed World for Research on Television in the Developing World, *Journal of Cross-Cultural Psychology*, 16(3) (1985), 263–288.

W. Wundt, *Elements of Folk Psychology* (New York: Macmillan, 1916).

Index